The For-Profit Hospital

THE FOR-PROFIT HOSPITAL

- ACCESS
- QUALITY
- TEACHING
- RESEARCH

Edited by
Richard McK. F. Southby, Ph.D.
Warren Greenberg, Ph.D.

The 1984 Harold and Jane Hirsh Symposium
The George Washington University—Battelle
Health Policies Series—1984

BATTELLE PRESS
Columbus • Richland

Printed in the United States of America.

Library of Congress Cataloging-in-Publication Data

Harold and Jane Hirsh Symposium (1984: Washington, D.C.)
The for-profit hospital.

(The George Washington University–Battelle health policy series)
Symposium held in Washington, D.C.
Includes bibliographies and index.
1. Hospitals, Proprietary–Congresses. 2. Hospital care–Congresses. 3. Hospitals, Teaching–Congresses. 4. Hospitals–Research–Congresses. 5. Hospitals, Proprietary–United States–Congresses. 6. Hospital care–United States–Congresses. 7. Hospitals, Teaching–United States–Congresses. 8. Hospitals–Research–United States–Congresses. I. Southby, Richard McK. F. II. Greenberg, Warren, 1943- . III. Title. IV. Series. [DNLM: 1. Delivery of Health Care–United States–Congresses. 2. Economics, Hospital–United States–Congresses. 3. Health Services Accessibility–United States–Congresses. 4. Hospitals–United States–Congressses. 5. Quality of Health Care–United States–Congresses. WX 157 H254f 1984
RA875,074H37 1984 362.1′1. 85–26729
ISBN 0–935470–24–7

Contents

Foreword: vii
Lloyd H. Elliott, *President,*
The George Washington University

Preface ix
Richard McK. F. Southby, Ph.D., &
Warren Greenberg, Ph.D.

Acknowledgments xv

TEACHING AND RESEARCH

Introductory Remarks: Teaching and Research 3
Ronald P. Kaufman, M.D.,
Vice President for Medical Affairs and Executive Dean of the School of Medicine and Health Sciences, The George Washington University, Washington, D.C.

A Case Study 7
Philip S. Birnbaum, M.S. in M.E.,
Dean of the Medical Center for Administrative Affairs and Professor of Health Services Administration, The George Washington University.

The Involvement of For-Profit Hospital Chains with Teaching and Research Institutions 19
Richard H. Egdahl, M.D.,
Director, Boston University Medical Center and the Center for Industry and Health Care.

The Implications for Teaching and Research 32
Ruth S. Hanft, M.A.,
Consultant in Health Policy Research, Washington, D.C.

Discussions—Teaching and Research 45

QUALITY

Introductory Remarks: Status on the Quality of Care ... 57
Kurt Darr, Sc.D., J.D., F.A.C.H.E.,
Professor, Department of Health Services Administration, The George Washington University

The Implications for Quality of Care 63
James P. LoGerfo, M.D., M.P.H.,
Professor of Medicine and Health Services, Co-Director, The Robert Wood Johnson Clinical Scholars Program, University of Washington, Schools of Medicine and Public Health & Community Medicine

How Does the Profit Motive Affect the Quality of Care? 76
Penelope C. Roeder,
Assistant Vice President
American Medical International, Inc., and
John H. Moxley III, M.D.,
Senior Vice President,
American Medical International, Inc.

Discussions—Quality 85

ACCESS

Introductory Remarks: Access to Health Care 101
Warren Greenberg, Ph.D.,
Associate Professor, Department of Health Services Administration, The George Washington University

The Impact of Investor Owned Hospitals on Access to Health Care 105
Robert A. Vraciu, Ph.D.,
Vice President, Strategic Planning & Research
Hospital Corp. of America and
Phyllis M. Virgil, M.P.A.
Manager, Strategic Planning,
Hospital Corp. of America

The Implications of Hospital Ownership on Access to Care 130
Stephen M. Shortell, Ph.D.
A. C. Buehler, *Distinguished Professor of Hospital and Health Services Management and Professor of Organization Behavior, J. L. Kellogg Graduate School of Management and Center for Health Services and Policy Research, Northwestern University, Evanston, Illinois*

Whither the Soul of Health Care? 143
Basil J. F. Mott, *Ph.D.*
Dean, School of Health Studies, University of New Hampshire

Discussions—Access 151

Index 159

Foreword

The establishment of the Hirsh Symposia by the Department of Health Services Administration at the George Washington University is a recent initiative which should have considerable impact on the debates about health policy issues in the United States for many years to come.

Careful attention has been given to the planning of these symposia to ensure that they will be very different from the usual types of conferences, meetings, or seminars. No more than thirty distinguished persons will be invited to each symposium to discuss a health policy topic which is of current concern and significance for the United States health system. By keeping the size of the group to a relatively small number, the participants should be able to engage in meaningful and constructive dialogues. Following each annual symposium the main papers presented will be published as a book and over the years these publications will make significant contributions to the analysis of policy issues confronting administrators, educators, patients, politicians, providers, researchers, students, and the general public.

This book, *The For-Profit Hospital: Access, Quality, Teaching and Research* is of special interest to this University at this time. As many will be aware, The George Washington University is in the process of negotiating the possible lease of the University Hospital to American Medical International, Inc. Similar negotiations, resulting in the lease or sale of university affiliated hospitals, have been occurring in different parts of the country and with a variety of health care corporations. The chapters of this book will be read with great interest by everyone at The George Washington University who is interested in the future of our hospital and the requirements for it to remain a leading institution for service, education, and research.

These symposia have been made possible by a generous annual grant from Dr. Harold Hirsh and his wife Jane. Doctor Hirsh is a distinguished physician and health lawyer in Washington, D.C., and has been a member of The George Washington University faculty for many years.

The Department of Health Services Administration, the School of Government and Business Administration, and the University are grateful for the generous financial support from Harold and Jane Hirsh and are delighted to name these symposia in their honor.

It is a pleasure for me to record the association of Battelle Human Affairs Research Centers with the University in the annual publication of this series. As a result of this collaboration, the ideas discussed at the Hirsh Symposia will reach a wide audience of interested persons throughout the United States.

Lloyd H. Elliott
President
The George Washington University

Preface

This book, *The For-Profit Hospital: Access, Quality, Teaching and Research* contains the papers presented at the 1984 Harold and Jane Hirsh Symposium. It is the first of an annual series sponsored by the Institute of Health Policy and Administration, within the Department of Health Services Administration at The George Washington University.

In line with the aim of these symposia of focusing on a health policy topic which is of current concern and significance for the United States health care system, the 1984 Hirsh Symposium discussed The Implications of The For-Profit Hospital in Health Care. There is no doubt that the role of the for-profit hospitals is attracting a great deal of attention in the health field at the present time. A distinguished group of presenters and participants came together in Washington, D.C., on October 3 and 4, 1984, and provided a wide variety of interesting and challenging viewpoints on this topic.

The symposium was divided into three main sections–The Implications for Teaching and Research; The Implications for the Quality of Health Care; and The Implications for Access to Health Care.

Dr. Ronald Kaufman, Vice President for Medical Affairs and Executive Dean of the School of Medicine and Health Sciences at The George Washington University, introduced and moderated the first section on teaching and research. In his introductory remarks, Dr. Kaufman drew attention to the fact that in spite of the dramatic growth of investor-owned hospital chains during the past decade, much of the "knowledge" about these organizations is based on little more than a series of myths. He suggested that in the future the contributions to education and research from the for-profit sector, while presently a small proportion of the total, may increase significantly.

Dr. Richard Egdahl, Director of the Boston University Medical Center and the Center for Industry and Health Care, spoke on the involvement of for-profit hospital chains with teaching and reasearch institutions. He considered the question of the potential benefits and conflicts between non-profit educational institutions and for-profit hospital chains. In his paper, Dr. Egdahl summarized five cases which looked at ownership and leasing, contract management, and direct grant arrangements by for-profit chains. Dr. Egdahl believes that it will be possible to have fruitful partnerships between for-profit companies and academic medical centers, if the arrangements are negotiated as tightly as possible before agreements are signed.

Ms. Ruth Hanft, Consultant in Health Policy Research, Washington, D.C., continued the examination of the implications for teaching and research. She stressed the need for collection of sufficient data to assess the effects of the involvement of the investor-owned firms in the health industry. Only then can the advantages and disadvantages be validated or rejected. Six myths about the relationships of for-profit hospitals and medical schools were presented and her elaboration of these myths provided some challenging questions for the field. Other areas covered by Ms. Hanft include considerations of the external environment, the possible motivations for the change from non-teaching to teaching status or the acquisition of a teaching hospital, the financing of medical and graduate medical education, and uncompensated and indigent care.

Dean Philip Birnbaum, Dean of the Medical Center for Administrative Affairs at The George Washington University, presented a case study based on the university's investigation of the possibility of the university developing an ownership or lease arrangement for the University Hospital with American Medical International, Inc. Dean Birnbaum outlined the objectives of the study and explained the special organizational structure of the medical center as it currently operates. The study has come to the conclusion that local control of the medical center, and not remote system-wide control, must be retained as an essential element of any agreement with American Medical International, Inc. Dean Birnbaum felt that these questions concerning the governance and decision-making processes would have been the same if the inquiry had focused on a not-for-profit chain rather than a for-profit organization.

Dr. Basil Mott, Dean of the School of Health Studies at the University of New Hampshire, challenged the participants in his luncheon address to review the changes which are occurring in the organization, delivery, financing, and provision of health services in the United States. One of his concerns is that in our eagerness to adapt to the changing environment as a means of survival, we risk transformations that could severely damage the American health care system. He expressed concern about the impact of these adaptations on moral responsibility and the charitable values which are reflected in the belief that health care is a right. Although business methods are of great benefit, and indeed, essential, to both non-profit and investor-owned institutions, he suggested that there may be a confusion of means and ends.

The second major section of the symposium examined the implications of for-profit status on the quality of care. Dr. Kurt Darr, Professor of Health Services Administration and of Health Care Sciences at The George Washington University, introduced and moderated this section. In his comments Dr. Darr recalled the prediction made twenty years ago in many graduate programs in hospital administration that by the 1970s there would be no proprietary hospitals. Rather than declining, the for-profit hospitals have exhibited a dramatic increase in recent years. He posed the question of incompatability between the profit motives and the delivery of high quality health care. At the other extreme there is the view that medical care is really no different than other service activities. Once again, concern was expressed about the paucity of data necessary to answer the questions relating to profit in health care.

Dr. James LoGerfo, Professor of Medicine and Health Services at the University of Washington, reviewed studies of quality in for-profit institutions and concluded that they are either outdated or that the variance is inadequately explained by the data. He suggested that organizations will assure themselves of profits either by moving to product or service lines which are profitable or by using cost-reduction stategies. In his concluding comments Dr. LoGerfo emphasized the significance of research, which demonstrated that greater physician involvement in management and governing board decisions was also linked with higher quality of care.

The second paper in this section asked how the profit motive affects the quality of care and was authored by Ms. Penelope Roeder, Assistant Vice President, and Dr. John Moxley, Senior Vice President of American Medical International, Inc. These authors, like Dr. LoGerfo, also stressed the role of the medical staff in determining the allocation of resources and the ramifications for the quality of care. They found no significant differences between the investor-owned and the not-for-profit hospitals as far as medical staff organization and involvement in decision making was concerned. Attention was also directed to the perceived impacts of the new prospective payment system.

The third section of the symposium concentrated on the implications of the for-profit hospital for access to health care. Dr. Warren Greenberg, Co-Editor of this book and Associate Professor of Health Services Administration at The George Washington University, outlined some of the economic assumptions of the behavior of for-profit and not-for-profit hospitals. He also provided an example from the health insurance industry which included the non-profit Blue Cross firms as well as the for-profit commerical carriers to illustrate the behavior of non-profit firms. In response to increasing pressures on their financial resources, the federal government and many state governments have recently imposed constraints on reimbursements to hospitals, in addition to encouraging increased competition in the system, as ways of containing health care costs.

Dr. Robert Vraciu, Vice President, Strategic Planning, and Research, and Ms. Phyllis Virgil, Coordinator of Strategic Planning of Hospital Corporation of America, provided evidence which supports the conclusion that investor-owned hospitals are comparable to the not-for-profit hospitals in relation to access to care. They emphasized that although the investor-owned hospitals are not the solution to access problems, neither are they the cause. In other words, ownership does not appear to determine the patterns of access to hospitals. They pointed to four policy questions which need to be answered if the access problems are to be resolved.

Dr. Stephen Shortell, A.C. Buehler Distinguished Professor of Hospital and Health Services Management at Northwestern University, made the second presentation to this section of the symposium. He offered some additional perspectives on the implications of hospital ownership on access to care. Recent evidence, according to Dr. Shortell, suggests that access to for-profit hospitals by the indigent is somewhat more restricted than access to non-profit hospitals. He provided eleven points which support his assertion that the United States as a nation has never faced up to the issue of making available a basic set of health services, however comprehensive or restrictive such a basic set may be. The access issue is much larger than merely a question of ownership differences. He also discussed the meaning of access, outlined three factors which have been shown to be associated with differences in access to care, summarized the state of existing knowledge about the relationship between hospital ownership forms and access to care, and finally posed some questions and made some recommendations for future investigations. Included in his paper is an interesting causal model of the dimensions of health services provision.

The For-Profit Hospital also includes the remarks of invited health policy makers, health care executives, and academics who commented on the papers of the primary contributors. These comments reflect the extent of the controversy surrounding teaching and research, quality of care, and access to care within the acute care hospital sector.

The reader will find that while the contributors to this volume have not answered all the complex health policy questions associated with the for-profit hospitals, they have achieved the following:

- Summarized the significant research in this field to date as it relates to the performance of the for-profit hospital system.
- Indentified gaps in our knowledge of this sector and its impact on the health system.
- Challenged many of the "myths" associated with the for-profit hospitals.
- Clarified our understanding of the comparative performance of the for-profit and not-for-profit hospitals in the health system.
- Posed questions which need to be addressed by researchers and policy makers if these problems are to be resolved.

RICHARD MCK. F. SOUTHBY, PH.D.
Professor and Chairman,
Department of Health Services Administration,
and Professor of Health Care Services
The George Washington University
Washington, D.C.

WARREN GREENBERG, PH.D.
Associate Professor,
Department of Health Services Administration
The George Washington University,
Washington, D.C.

Acknowledgements

We are particularly grateful to the following individuals for their assistance in preparing this book for publication. Ms. Laurie Havens, Graduate Student and Research Assistant in the Department of Health Services Administration, who has done much of the detailed editing and indexing of the papers; Mrs. Helen Klepac, Office Supervisor, Department of Health Services Administration, for her administrative support at the time of the symposium and coordinating the typing of the papers; Mr. Syed Hossain, Senior Word Processing Operator, Department of Health Services Administration and Ms. Joyce Smith, Administrative Secretary, Battelle Human Affairs Research Centers, for successfully converting the drafts into the final typed versions for word processing; Dr. Bryan Luce, Senior Research Scientist, Battelle Human Affairs Research Centers, who has been our primary contact with Battelle as the publishers of this new annual health policy series; and Mr. Joseph Sheldrick, Manager, and Mr. Morrie Helitzer, Consulting Publisher, Battelle Press, who have guided us through the maze of practicalities in the production of this volume.

Teaching and Research

RONALD P. KAUFMAN, M.D.
Vice President for Medical Affairs and Executive Dean of the School of Medicine and Health Sciences, The George Washington University, Washington, D.C.

Introductory Remarks: Teaching and Research

There has been a dramatic emergence during the past decade of investor-owned hospital chains. Equally dramatic and perhaps just as surprising, is how little is truly known about these for-profit chains and how much of what is "known" is based primarily on the conventional wisdom of the moment, much of which is the result of intrinsic biases. Even the ways in which we refer to for-profit hospital groups reflect our prejudices. For instance, proprietary, for-profit, and investor-owned all convey more than a subliminal message to the audience.

This session addresses the implications for teaching and research in for-profit hospitals. Before we begin, however, permit me to present some data and to react to certain myths and "givens." First, it is frequently stated that by around 1990, 20 percent of hospital beds will be in for-profit chains. This prediction, of course, requires an interpretive definition of what comprises an investor-owned hospital group.

Donald S. McNaughton (1981), of the Hospital Corporation of America, defines such a group as private companies that own or manage, for others, a multiple number of hospitals and are themselves owned by stockholders. He further states that such companies currently account for more than 800 hospitals, or approximately 14 percent of the nation's 5,800 short-term, acute care community hospitals. They also account for approximately ten percent of hospital beds and these investor-owned groups are growing at a rate of approximately 15 percent per year.

On the other hand, Dan Ermann and Jon Gabel (1984), in their review of multi-hospital systems, used a different definition. They grouped together, under the term multi-hospital systems, for-profits and not-for-profits. They then defined such a system as two or more hospitals that are owned, managed, or leased by a single organization. According to Ermann and Gabel (1984), 36 percent of the nation's hospital beds belonged to such organizations. Based on their broad definition, Ermann and Gabel found that the average annual growth rate since 1978 has been approximately 3.5 percent, whether measuring the number of multi-hospital systems, the number of hospital beds, or the percentage of U.S. community hospitals in such systems. There does not seem to be any clear pattern of differences in the rate of growth between for-profit and not-for-profit systems. This very modest growth has occurred in the supportive climate of a retrospective cost-based reimbursement system. How the change in reimbursement to prospective pricing will affect the situation is speculative at best.

The second topic I wish to address is that investor-owned hospitals somehow modify medical practice by selection and influence of their medical staffs. Recent data from the American Medical Association (1983), indicate that only one out of every seven physicians admits patients primarily to proprietary hospitals. The data also indicate that there is little difference in the distribution of medical and surgical specialties between proprietary and non-proprietary hospitals and that physician practice income is slightly greater for physicians who practice primarily in non-proprietary hospitals. The differences between physicians whose principal privileges are in proprietary versus non-proprietary hospitals are very small.

On the average, proprietary hospitals have larger medical staffs and more board-certified medical specialists per 100 beds than non-proprietary hospitals. Furthermore, it does not appear that proprietary hospital ownership has adversely restricted physicians' clinical discretion. In sum, it seems difficult to assume from this limited data that proprietary hospitals select their medical staffs for Machiavellian purposes.

My intent is not to condemn or condone either sector but rather to emphasize my belief that many so-called facts are actually myths based on very soft and insufficient data; that very few good studies are available; and that considering the rapidly changing economic environment, this subject is ripe for solid research.

As a further prologue, let me present some very simple data that I have quickly collated (AAMC, 1982). In 1980, there were approximately 7,000 short-term, acute care hospitals. Around 800 are for-profit. Some 330 are members of the Council of Teaching Hospitals, and, of these, approximately 250 are non-profit, with the remainder being government-owned. For-profits cannot be members of the Council of Teaching Hospitals. The vast majority of undergraduate and graduate medical education takes place in members of the Council of Teaching Hospitals. Therefore, in rough numbers, some five percent of the acute care, short-term hospitals are responsible for well over 90 percent of the medical education in this country. A very quick and superficial review of for-profit hospitals, using the Directory of Accredited Residency Programs (1984-1985), reveals a total of 18 in 1983 with a medical school affiliation, a linkage to graduate medical education, or both. In other words, two percent (18/800) of the for-profits are involved in some graduate medical education program. Therefore, it seems that for-profit versus not-for-profit may well be a phantom issue, since only a small percentage of all hospitals have traditionally carried the major medical education burden. It was this realization, purposefully intermixed with the severity and intensity-of-care issue, which lead the Association of American Medical Colleges to lobby successfully to include both a direct and indirect pass-through for medical education under the diagnosis-related groups (DRG) prospective payment plan. It has been estimated by the Office of Management and Budget, among others, that this will cost the Medicare Hospital Trust Fund well over three billion dollars. For this and other reasons, the Medicare Advisory Council and a number of congressmen and senators have suggested that such a payment from the Medicare Hospital Trust Fund is inappropriate and that some other mechanism for funding medical education should be found. Any such action would severely disrupt the entire infrastructure of support for both undergraduate and graduate medical education.

There are no firm data on research in the investor-owned hospital sector. In fact, it was only recently that for-profit companies were eligible to receive grants from the National Institutes of Health. In my view, however, perhaps more significant than data was the choice of Dr. William DeVries (of the artificial heart fame) to leave the University of Utah to join the Humana Heart Institute to establish a heart-replacement program and continue his research (Blue Sheet, 1984). The Vice President for Health Sciences at the University of Utah stated that the University could not realistically compete with Humana's ability to support such research and its practical application. Whether this is an isolated incident or a forecast of things to come, only time will tell.

Perhaps as society's inclination to fund health care research and development decreases, investment from the for-profit sector will increase. David A. Jones, Chairman of the Board of Humana, Donald S. McNaughton, Chairman of the Board of Hospital Corporation of America, and Royce Diener, Chairman of the Board of American Medical International (1984), have emphatically stated that the future of their segment of the health care delivery system is dependent on the continued improvement and growth of the system, which requires an investment in education and research. Whether this will be accomplished independently by investor-owned chains or in association with academic health science centers remains to be seen.

Perhaps the key issue is whether the requirement to earn a reasonable profit, rightly an expectation of investors, creates such a major divergence in goals from 501(C)3 organizations that joint ventures or independent investments in research and education are inappropriate. In any event, the short but dramatic history of the for-profit hospital industry strengthens the notion that they are here to stay. The question is: What impact will they have on the education and research environment, which has been one of the major strengths of the American health care system?

REFERENCES

Association of American Medical Colleges. "A Description of Teaching Hospital Characteristics." December 1982.

American Medical Association. *Directory of Residency Training Programs Accredited by the Accredation Council for Graduate Medical Education.* Chicago: AMA, 1984.

American Medical Association. *Socio-economic Monitoring Systems,* 2(8), November 1983.

Diener, Royce. "Strategy and Structure Health Care Management in a Time of Change." Montgomery Dorsey Symposium, July 13, 1984.

Ermann, Dan and Gabel, Jon. "Multihospital Systems: Issues and Empirical Findings." *Health Affairs* 3(1):50–64, Spring 1984.

FDA Reports. *The Blue Sheet,* August 8, 1984.

McNaughton, Donald S. "Development of Investor-Owned Hospital Groups and Implications for Academic Centers." Paper presented at the Annual Meeting of the Association of Academic Medical Centers, November 3, 1981.

PHILIP S. BIRNBAUM, M.S. in M.E.
Dean of the Medical Center for Administrative Affairs and Professor of Health Services Administration, The George Washington University, Washington, D.C.

A Case Study

The theme of this conference, raising as it does the possibility of partnership between business and the academic health center, arouses strong feelings among many in academic medicine. The very concept of interaction between medical schools or academic health centers and the investor-owned sector is anathema to those who believe that there are irreconcilable differences between the not-for-profit and the for-profit sectors and that seeds of discord are contained in relationships between the two in health care. Arnold Relman, from the podium of the *New England Journal of Medicine,* became an eloquent spokesman for this group early in 1980, when he coined the phrase "medical-industrial complex." His colleagues at Harvard Medical School indicated their general agreement with him (Tosteson, 1983) when they rejected a proposed sale by the Massachusetts General Hospital (MGH) of its McLean facility to the Hospital Corporation of America (HCA). Nevertheless, in his letter to Dean Tosteson acknowledging the Harvard faculty's recommendation against the proposal, Francis Burr, Chairman of the Board of MGH, clearly noted that the status quo could not be maintained (Burr, 1983). At present, conversations continue between MGH and HCA on the McLean facility (Burr, 1984).

There are a number of relationships between for-profit hospitals and medical schools. For example, Humana, Inc. leases the hospital which serves as the primary teaching site for the medical school of the University of Louisville. Kmetz (1984) has described the background of a combined operating and capital deficit which eventually led to the negotiation of the lease. He noted that specific efforts were made during the discussions to address the frequently raised issue of indigent care and academic need. The lease agreement is of too short a duration for meaningful evaluation, but, by examining the relationship and deciding to enter into it, the officials of the state, county, hospital, and the University of Louisville indicated a willingness to explore this alternative solution to their problem. At Creighton University, American Medical International (AMI) has become involved in medical education by purchasing St. Joseph's Hospital, the primary teaching hospital for the Creighton University School of Medicine. The George Washington University (GWU) Medical Center foresaw difficulty in capital formation – much as at MGH – and decided to explore the investor-owned sector; there will undoubtedly be others.

This paper discusses the study underway at GWU on the possibility of an interaction with a proprietary health care chain, specifically AMI. It reviews the purpose of (or perhaps) the philosophy behind undertaking the study in the form that it is and the method by which it has progressed. A report of the issues and a current proposed resolution of some of these issues is included. The paper closes with some speculation on the implications for the study if a relationship with a not-for-profit chain rather than a for-profit chain had been under consideration.

The objectives of the study were:

1. To determine the requirements of a structure that would safeguard the University's need to ensure appropriate control of the resources supporting the missions of educational (at undergraduate and graduate levels), research, and patient care (as a community service).
2. To evaluate, in terms of the requirements determined in the first step, the hospital's operating and capital status, current and prospective consumer (patient) profiles, current and prospective resource requirements to meet the mission needs, and environmental factors.
3. To determine and describe accurately the roles, responsibilities, and relationships of academic departments and support elements to be included in any agreement between GWU and AMI. This involves review of current AMI operations in situations most similar to the GWU circumstances and the determination of AMI policies and procedures that must be specifically addressed.

4. To design an agreement that addresses the administrative governance structure required to satisfy the needs of the University's programs with adequate safeguards to protect the integrity of these programs while meeting the needs of AMI.
5. To develop a detailed implementation plan for the agreement reached, including approval by appropriate faculty and governing bodies.

As the study proceeded, Item 2 became routine, and since fiscal aspects are not within the scope of this paper, it will not be discussed further. Items 1, 3, and 4 form the framework around which the study was built, while Item 5 is only a brief outline indicating a negotiating process if all preceding conditions can be satisfactorily resolved.

The organizational structure at GWU (Figure 1) is part of the background of the study. There is a single corporate entity, the University, with a single board of trustees. The Medical Center is administered by Dr. Ronald Kaufman, who carries the dual title of University Vice President for Medical Affairs and Executive Dean of the Medical Center. He is assisted by three deans of the Medical Center: Dr. L. T. Bowles (Academic Affairs), Dr. Dennis O'Leary (Clinical Affairs), and myself (Administrative Affairs). These three are program coordinators with no line authority over any of the academic departments. The Vice President and the deans form, in effect, a management committee (the Office of the Vice President for Medical Affairs [OVPMA]), with total control over all the assets of the Medical Center, subject only to approval by the President of the University and the Board of Trustees. Senior non-academic staff members, such as the Director of Financial Services, serve the entire Medical Center–school, hospital, and group practice. The Medical Center budget, about $200 million for this year, is about 25 per cent greater than the sum of the budgets of all the other components of the University and is submitted separately to the Board. The fiscal relationships between the Medical Center and the remainder of the University are such that OVPMA has, for all practical purposes, complete discretion within the approved total budget.

With the strong support of GWU's President and Board of Trustees Executive Committee, exploratory discussions with Dr. John Moxley, Vice-President for Strategic Planning, acting on behalf of AMI, were entered into in mid-1983. Moxley's experience in academic medicine made such conversations very easy to pursue, and he received from the Board of AMI full support in entering into

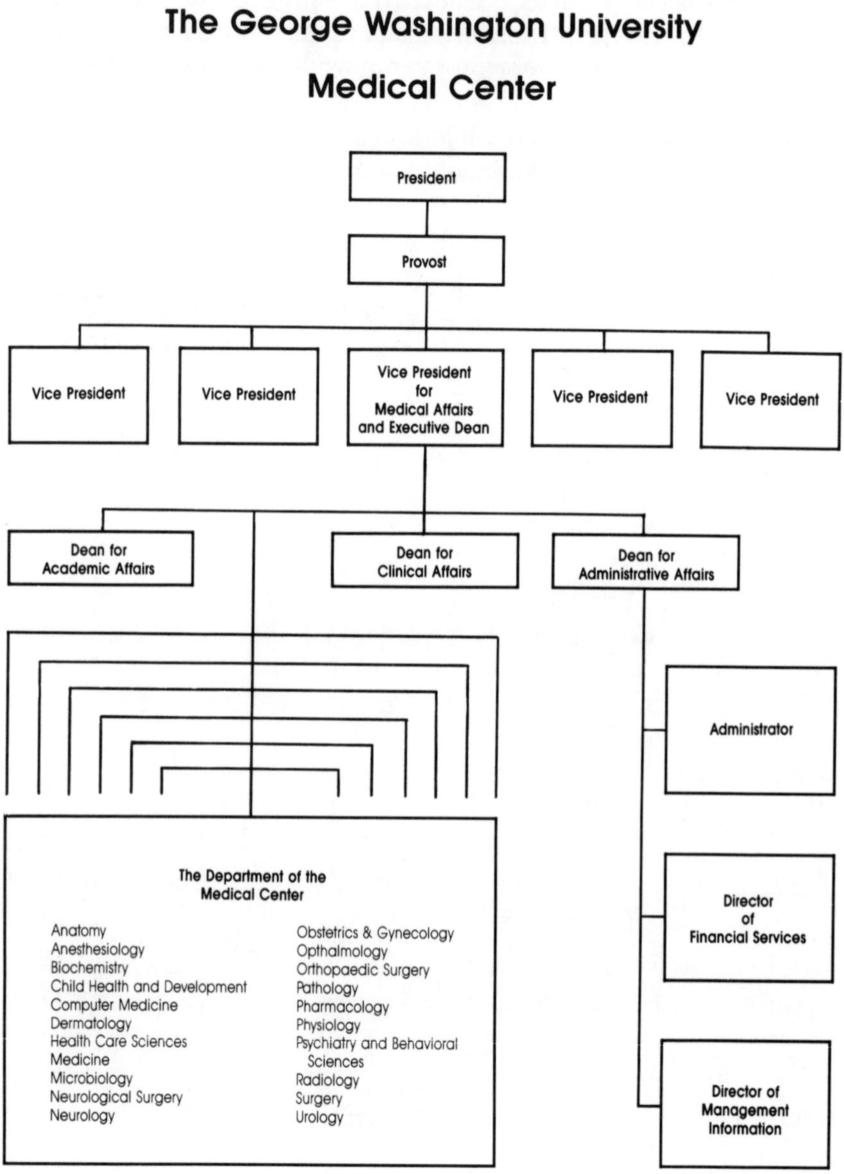

FIGURE 1. The George Washington University Organizational Structure.

these explorations. It is not an exaggeration to say that GWU's selection of AMI as the proprietary health care organization was heavily influenced by Moxley's presence at AMI's corporate level and AMI's assignment of him as the primary contact. After some preliminary discussions and with agreement that this study, unlike the behind-the-scenes negotiations that had taken place in other institutions, would be as public as feasible and would concentrate on examining the issues openly, approval to proceed was received from the two boards. No commitment was made as to whether there would be a relationship and, if there were, whether it would be consummated with AMI. It also was agreed that participation by the GWU Medical Center constituencies would be as broadly representative as feasible.

It was hoped that some of the benefits to GWU of a relationship with the for-profit sector would also be advantageous to the community. For instance, George Washington University would be maintained as a strong contributor to academic health care programs and to public health care needs. The physical structure of the hospital would be improved and technology advanced so as to enhance public access to hospital services. New management structures would be developed that would offer more rapid implementation of Medical Center and hospital programs and services and that would provide students with excellent medical education and expanded health care opportunities. Finally, the study would be published as a demonstration guide for others seeking alternatives and solutions to the changing health care environment.

To develop a series of options that could be examined in light of the relevant issues, a steering advisory committee was formed comprised of the Vice President for Medical Affairs, the three Medical Center deans, Moxley, and a vice president for development at AMI. I served as project director or principal investigator. In addition, four formal working groups were established. One, chaired by Dr. Bowles, examined education and research. The second group, chaired by Dr. O'Leary, investigated clinical affairs. The third group was established under the Administrator of the Medical Center, Michael Barch, to review the implications for hospital operations and interaction with other elements of the Medical Center and the University. The fourth group, which was chaired by Thomas Carroll, Director of Financial Services for the Medical Center, reviewed the implications of various fiscal options for a relationship between AMI and GWU.

It was our original plan that the working groups would have significant representation from AMI and that after the initial phase of issue definition, the same working groups would address themselves to devising solutions to the problems enunciated in the first phase. The working groups, which were represented full-time and voluntary faculty, house staff, medical students, nurses, and administrative personnel, were very enthusiastic in their discussions, debates, and review of the literature and of the overall potential of a relationship between AMI and GWU. By late May, it had become apparent that the issue-definition phase was nearing completion. Although AMI staff members had occasionally been present at meetings of the working groups, and while Moxley and others at AMI had received minutes of each group's meetings, it was apparent that the distance separating AMI corporate headquarters (Beverly Hills) from the GWU campus (Washington, D.C.) had precluded the degree of participation by AMI staff that GWU had originally contemplated. It was therefore agreed to revise the plan in order to remain within the original January 1985 time frame for the study. In brief, the results of the issue-definition phase would be supplied to AMI, and AMI, in turn, would propose solutions to these issues. Because of the modest participation by AMI in Phase I, it was agreed that there would be similar limited participation by GWU as AMI developed its response. The AMI response was to be in the form of one or more possible relationship models – purchase, lease, or other arrangements – and a governance structure that together would appropriately address the identified requirements.

As the working groups progressed during Phase I, general concerns of the various constituencies were brought into the open to elicit the reactions of other constituencies in addition to the occasional AMI representative. During the course of three to six meetings in a three-month period, the undifferentiated anxiety-based issues were refined into concrete concerns. In the education and research group, for example, general statements on the need to protect academic freedom, including freedom of research and access to facilities for education and research, tended to be translated into concerns about numbers of services, bed allocations, house staff positions, and designation of chiefs of services. In the clinical affairs group, the anxieties of voluntary and full-time physicians concerning access to the hospital and continuity of support services became specific questions of control, as did the proposed role of the nursing services. As had been expected, the groups on hospital operations and financial services tended to be reactive in contrast to the proactive operations of the other two groups. They supplied data in response to requests from AMI but also generated lists of subjects about what information would be necessary and what actions would be required to be taken under any change in existing hospital operating status. Examples ranged from the need to develop a balance sheet separate from the integrated balance sheet used at present by the University to concern over the licensing provisions of the District of Columbia and the employment status of the hospital's non-academic staff.

Analysis of these issues led to the observation that organizational locus or site of control might be the key to a solution. Thus, issues were proposed to AMI in three groups. The first group were those matters that from the standpoint of GWU could not be negotiated. The second group comprised those issues about which we felt any relationship had to provide clear-cut and mutually satisfactory commitments. The third group became a laundry list of those issues that were identified as requiring attention but about which neither commitment nor predetermined definition was considered necessary.

Under Group 1 came the following four major categories: (1) the authority to specify process and to make decisions on medical staff membership; the services to be provided within the University Hospital; the selection of specific major items of diagnostic and therapeutic equipment within fund limits set by AMI after consultation with GWU; the selection of staffing patterns regarding nurses, technical support staff, and other care-giver personnel; the assignment of priority operating room time and admitting and facility access; and the assignment of space utilization; (2) the direct access of the OVPMA to AMI's corporate level regardless of any regional or other AMI organizational structure; (3) prior approval of affiliations involving the hospital or involving public identification with GWU; and (4) policy concerning patient admissions (i.e., financial class, diagnosis, or admitting physician). Comparison of these four major categories with the issues defined by the working groups indicates that the major concerns of each group are contained within these categories.

Under Group 2 came commitments that AMI would have to specify but about which GWU had no requirements for either control or preselected outcomes. These included the role and direction of the nursing service, establishment of services in the hospital that might compete with services offered by the GWU faculty group practice, the method of expressing AMI's corporate identity (i.e., might the hospital's name be changed?), the relationship of GWU to other AMI operations in the sense of forming an integrated system, and the support of faculty salary positions related to hospital duties such as house staff supervision, administrative duties, and committee service.

Group 3 formed a "laundry list" of 12 items not considered to be all-inclusive. Among these were relationships with the Federal and D.C. governments; buy-back provisions or other termination parameters; communications interactions with, say, the telephone system; union relationships, since GWU has union contracts with certain groups of its employees in the University and the hospital; long-term capital needs; security and parking services; and management information systems.

These issues were forwarded to AMI, which had proposed organizational and governance structures and relationship options, as was agreed. AMI staff members assigned from the various operating groups at the Beverly Hills office had acquired significant operating data and had made investigations of applicable regulatory or statutory requirements while they designed the response. GWU's input into this process had been largely through the furnishing of data as requested and through limited participation in working sessions at the Beverly Hills AMI headquarters.

AMI found no policy impediment to acceptance of the control conditions posed by GWU. As a general approach, there has been mutual agreement that the process should be described not in terms of AMI's standard approach of buying a hospital but in terms of the unique opportunity to participate in an academic health center. These discussions, in turn, have led to examination of a broadening relationship between the Medical Center and AMI that might include other AMI facilities.

The design of a governance or administrative structure that would maintain the strong, centrally integrated nature of GWU's current academic health center, yet provide AMI with that degree of input and control that would be appropriate to any significant involvement on its part, was more difficult.

The structure that has been provisionally developed and that seems to provide GWU with sufficient control to satisfy its perceived needs hinges on the development of the board that would direct the hospital. As currently designed (Figure 2), this board would consist of the four members of the existing OVPMA at GWU and three members designated by and representing AMI. It would exercise full authority for the hospital within operating and capital budget constraints applied by AMI. The magnitude of the financial resources made available might become the sticking point, either at the beginning of negotiations or, if an agreement were consummated, at some

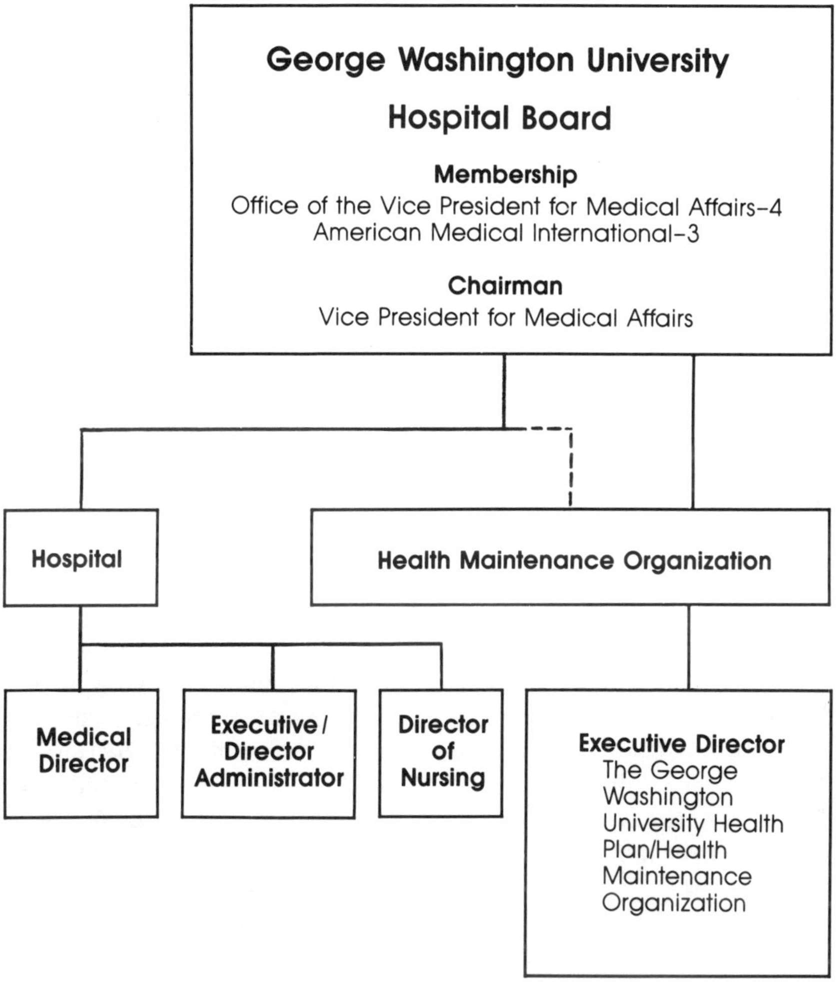

FIGURE 2. Proposed Organization Structure and Governance.

future point. Accordingly, some buy-out or buy-back provisions will be included in any agreement. AMI has indicated no intention of changing the structure of the nursing service or of interfering in any of the operational linkages that currently bind the University Hospital to the Medical Center. Although such Medical Center staff members as the Administrator and the Director of Financial Services are primarily involved in hospital operations, they also are involved in support of the school, the faculty group practice (MFA), and the Medical Center (central) administration. Current AMI proposals envision these individuals continuing to perform their existing functions as AMI employees, with their services purchased by the University on a time-and-effort basis in a manner similar to the current cost distribution of their salaries.

An interesting expansion of the potential relationship proposed by AMI involves the creation of a GWU-based regional network that would include, under the authority of the Board established for control of the hospital, the control of other AMI functions in the general geographic region in which the University Hospital and its Medical Center would become the hub. It is not possible at this time to forecast whether these proposals will surmount all the difficulties that may be perceived. Other academic health centers more traditionally organized than GWU might find the process much easier and much less fraught with organizational problems. Similarly, as the working groups reconvene to review the AMI-proposed structure, issues not yet surfaced may be found, or significant objections to the proposed solutions may be raised. Throughout this study, the input from the working groups has been evaluated as the Office of the Vice President prepares to make recommendations to the Board of Trustees.

The five objectives of this study were stated earlier in this paper. The first three have been achieved through the activities of the working groups and the transmission of necessary data between GWU and AMI. The last two objectives (i.e., the design of an agreement and the development of a detailed implementation plan) are not yet complete. The study, which had completed its first four objectives, was presented to the University Board of Trustees in January 1985. The fifth objective will probably be achieved only in outline form, since the successful completion of the study does not presage the successful completion of financial negotiations.

As the position is now evaluated, a significant part of the original objectives has been accomplished and has been faithful to the concept of a study to address issues versus a negotiation of price and value. What has emerged might be characterized as a definition of site of control. A process that permits the academic leadership of the health center to continue to decide those issues that have been identified as critical has been designed. The proprietary organization has indicated the acceptability of the solution. This may serve as a summary report of current status.

I would like to speculate on any differences in our study (in terms of objective, process, or outcome) had GWU's focus been on a relationship with a not-for-profit entity rather than with AMI. The word speculate is accurate, for there are no firm data to support the following views, nor do they represent the views of my colleagues or study participants.

I believe that from the start, the very concept of a study might not have emerged had we considered discussions with a not-for-profit entity. Questions raised both by perceived differences in objectives and by a fear that the values of our academic community were not compatible with the objectives of the investor-owned sector probably would not have surfaced. On the other hand, normal anxiety in the face of change would have been similar and efforts by various groups to safeguard or even improve their positions in terms of control, or in economic terms, might have been much the same. I suggest, however, that the rhetoric would have been very different. In contemplating investor-ownership, individuals and groups could maneuver for their own ends under the cover of concern for system values. Such terms might not have been useful in contemplating a not-for-profit partner. It seems more likely that negotiations for a specific relationship might have been the opening step, with issues of locus of control coming to light during the process.

Nevertheless, I believe that the real issues would have been the same. Implications for quantity and quality of education and research (as well as patient care) would have translated into control questions without regard to the nature or even the mission of the prospective partner. Voluntary faculty would have perceived on one hand an emerging or potential threat to its access to the hospital and on the other hand a chance to enhance its role and influence on the decision-making governance structure. Full-time faculty might have been on guard against a "central-office" approach to determining the size of residency programs or might have been concerned about its role in technology-acquisition decisions. At the level of the health care center, mechanisms to interface the hospital into health center needs would still have been of concern.

I believe that public perceptions would also have been different. There would have been little concern over possible implications for care of the economically disadvantaged. In reality, however, there has been little or no evidence of public concern despite full public disclosure. This does not mean that there will be no reaction to the study when it is published nor to any negotiations that might follow. But such reaction will be addressed to the patient care issue, and since the purpose of this paper is to look at implications for education and research, I will not pursue further the public aspects.

The study has come to the proposed solution of retaining the authority of the Medical Center's existing governance and decision-making structure and process, and I do not believe a different solution would have been found if a not-for-profit chain had been involved. The issue was local, goal-congruent control, not remote, system-wide, goal-oriented control, and was not directly affected by judgments as to the propriety of the goals, especially if the solution protects local autonomy in decisions.

REFERENCES

Burr, F. H. Letter to D. C. Tosteson, Dean, Harvard Medical School, November 1, 1983.

Burr, F. H. Personal Correspondence with Author, August/September, 1984.

Kmetz, Donald. "Investor-Owned Corporations and the Teaching Hospital." Unpublished paper presented at the Council of Teaching Hospitals Meeting, May, 1984.

Relman, A. S. "The New Medical-Industrial Complex." *The New England Journal of Medicine*, 303(17):963–970, October 23, 1980.

Tosteson, D. C. Letter to the Faculty of Medicine, Harvard Medical School, November 1, 1983.

RICHARD H. EGDAHL, M.D.
*Director,
Boston University Medical Center
and The Center for Industry and Health Care*

The Involvement of For-Profit Hospital Chains With Teaching and Research Institutions

Originally, most for-profit hospital chains were small and located in relatively affluent communities. Over the past several years however, an explosive growth of such institutions has occurred. The for-profit chains have moved into larger urban areas with medical schools and their associated teaching hospitals. The schools and teaching hospitals have worked out–and are expanding–a wide range of legal and economic ties. The for-profit chains have activated–or were negotiating as of October, 1984–ownership, leasing, management, and joint venture arrangements with teaching hospitals (both tertiary care-oriented university hospitals and affiliated community hospitals) and are providing grants for research projects to university medical schools.

The following discussion is based on a perspective that acknowledges both the fact and the legitimacy of the profit-seeking corporation's role in health care. Profit can be a powerful engine for the efficient operation of health care institutions, a useful incentive for cost control and improved performance, and a stimulus for raising patient satisfaction with the health care provided. But even among those who acknowledge the potential benefits of ties between educational institutions and for-profit chains, there is concern about close links between groups with the seemingly disparate goals of return on equity to shareholders and the promotion of education and research. Under what circumstances are these goals competitive and under what circumstances are they supportive of each other? What potential dangers and possible conflicts of interest do medical schools and their associated teaching hospitals face in forming financial and management ties with for-profit corporations? Under what conditions will a for-profit partner, acting on economic motives, seek to pull out of an arrangement, and what protection will the non-profit partner have? Finally, what are the risks or potential drawbacks of linkages between for-profit and educational institutions?

The relationship between for-profit hospital companies and academic medical centers is in a state of flux. Indeed, many changes will occur over the next few months and years. The tremendous upward pressures on health care costs and, in particular, the financial problems of teaching hospitals make probable a continuing evolution of complex linkages between academic medical centers and cash-rich for-profit hospital chains. Described herein are examples of these cooperative ventures and some of the problems and rewards that may result in terms of the effect of for-profit involvement on medical student education and residency training, as well as on basic and health care research. The primary point of emphasis relates to the range of direct involvement of for-profit hospital chains with academic medical centers.

The potential range of involvement between for-profit hospital corporations and teaching and research and of the degree of control the investor-owned company wields is broad. At one extreme, a for-profit company may own and support a teaching and/or research institution, either as an independent entity or, more commonly, with ties to an existing academic medical center. At the other extreme, the company may offer to fund specific research projects or teaching programs in existing institutions in a manner not significantly different from traditional governmental or private grant procedures. Between the two extremes – ownership and limited financial support – lie a variety of arrangements – joint ventures, management contracts, leasing – through which the for-profit company participates in the operation of academic medical centers.

At least in theory, numerous benefits accrue to both the academic centers and companies joining in these arrangements. The former may receive a vital new supply of funds: dollars for building and research, money for the salaries of both faculty and non-academic personnel, and the like. They may obtain access to the generally well-reputed management of the for-profit companies, their marketing skills, and their operational efficiencies. Furthermore, the for-profit chains, with their regional (and sometimes national) distribution of services, have extensive patient data bases that may be of use in academic research and training.

The for-profit companies, in turn, also benefit in the cooperative ventures. As in any large-scale real estate or capital property transaction, there is the opportunity for substantial tax benefits. Companies hope that in the teaching/research institution, they have a potentially profitable new line of business and access to consultation with academic faculty. The prestige involved in acquiring or working with a highly respected academic center can be an important positioning point–a chance to increase credibility with potential patients in all the chain's member hospitals. An impressive academic institution can serve as a "flagship" for a for-profit chain, a citadel for the chain's professional reputation, and a demonstration of the chain's commitment to its headquarters city or another city with an outstanding clinical reputation.

The flagship concept has some beneficial implications for the academic partner, too. To the extent that a flagship is seen (in what may be an oversimplification) as a kind of prestigious loss leader, there is greater incentive for the company to make decisions about the institution that are not based solely on profitability. Thus, more money than might otherwise be made available for teaching and research is spent to bolster the company's image. In hard times, a company might be more prone to continue to support a flagship institution if its decision were not based purely on economics.

In listing the advantages of cooperation between the for-profit company and the academic medical center, it should be noted that the potential benefits are not necessarily in conflict, especially if both institutions are involved in a phase of growth and increasing revenues. It is primarily when the market slumps or when the particular benefits of an arrangement start to fade that the interests of the partners may begin to diverge.

The greatest potential disadvantage to the academic medical center occurs when the for-profit chain decides to withdraw from the arrangement or not to renew a lease or insists that the academic partner or a third party buy out the for-profit company's equity. Would the academic partner have enough financial and management resources to keep an institution going? Would it have grown too dependent on the for-profit company's involvement to go it alone? Are there ways the for-profit partner could "milk" an institution over the short-term, reducing its economic viability, and then withdraw? Short of actual withdrawal, are there pressures that might entice a for-profit entity to alter the patient mix or treatment patterns of patients in ways that undermine the teaching and research goals of the institution?

The for-profit partner could also suffer in arrangements that turn sour. In addition to those factors that could make any hospital operation unsound, there are some special elements at work in the teaching hospital situation. These include the possible clinical inefficiency of physicians in an academic medical center, which reduces the revenue produced by these doctors. Furthermore, if the company started to lose money in a relationship, its expected–and economically rational–response might lead to harmful publicity for it.

These general recurring risks and benefits of cooperative ventures should be kept in mind as some of the specifics of current developments are examined.

CASES

A. Ownership of a Free-Standing Research-Oriented Hospital by a For-Profit Chain

Humana, Inc., located in Louisville, Kentucky, is an example of a for-profit corporation that wholly owns an independent clinical, research-oriented entity. This situation affords the corporation the highest degree of control. Humana operates the 484-bed Humana Hospital-Audubon, home of the Humana Heart Institute, and a group of other Centers of Excellence that it is establishing (New York Times 1984 a, b, c; Clark, 1984). These research centers will operate separately from Humana Hospital University, which the chain leases from the University of Louisville.

The Humana Heart Institute was established in 1983 under the guidance of cardiovascular surgeon Dr. Allan Lansing. In 1984, Lansing successfully lured to the institute Dr. William C. DeVries, of the University of Utah. DeVries had expressed frustration with the University of Utah's approval procedures in regard to implant operations. Humana, in addition to increasing DeVries' salary, also pledged to provide funding for facilities and patient care for 100 artificial heart implants, a financial package that the University of Utah could not possibly match. DeVries and Lansing are private practicing physicians involved in clinical investigation. According to Humana's chairman, David Jones, the corporation not only has ample revenue to support such research but, due to its business efficiencies, can do so at lower cost than non-profit institutions.

The Humana Hospital-Audubon example raises some troubling issues and some thorny possibilities for conflict of interest. Both the University of Utah and Humana own equity in Symbion, the company that manufactures the artificial heart. DeVries is a shareholder and had been asked by the University of Utah to divest himself of his stock. We thus find a situation where a for-profit company, seeking to become the principal center for heart implant operations, hires away from a university a doctor who owns equity in the product he is inserting.

The Institutional Review Board is designed to protect the interests of patients in such ethical tangles, required of entities receiving federal funds for human experimentation. It was the purportedly slow procedures of this board at the University of Utah that are said to have prompted DeVries' move. At Humana, he deals with a board no doubt drawing its membership largely from Humana employees and leaders in the community. Whether such a board can successfully operate without prejudice in this situation is problematic. The impact of an institution dominant in a line of research, owned by a for-profit entity with a financial interest in the clinical application of the research, remains to be seen. At the least, the situation frames some complex ethical issues.

B. Acquisition of a University Hospital by a For-Profit Hospital Chain

In Omaha, Nebraska, American Medical International, Inc. (AMI), a hospital chain based in southern California, has brought about a striking new development in for-profit expansion, the outright acquisition of an existing university teaching hospital (FAH Review, 1984). AMI has agreed to buy, for approximately $100 million, St. Joseph's Hospital, the 539-bed teaching and tertiary care facility of Creighton University. AMI has a $2.2 billion revenue base and a multi-hospital system containing more than 130 facilities. Under the specific binding terms of the purchase agreement, AMI will operate St. Joseph's as a full-service teaching center for Creighton University and invest the resources necessary to position St. Joseph as the company's flagship and hub facility in the central Midwest. Although ownership of the hospital will lie clearly with AMI, a governing hospital board with "policy-making responsibility" will be established and will equally represent physicians, community and

Boys Town (long connected with St. Joseph's) representatives, university faculty/administrative representatives, and AMI personnel.

The jointly staffed board is a recurrent feature of arrangements between for-profit chains and academic medical centers. How it will handle conflicts with AMI, when legal ownership and fiscal control lie with the corporation, will be an important aspect of the St. Joseph's venture.

In addition to committing itself to financial support of current hospital programs, both clinical and academic, AMI has pledged to maintain the "spiritual mission" of the hospital and the Jesuit-run university. As Creighton's president, the Rev. Michael Morrison, S. J., said in an AMI press release, dated June 5, 1984:

> By the specific commitment in the agreement to perpetuate the catholicity and health services education roles of our primary teaching hospital, AMI demonstrates determination to support Creighton's traditional mission. We believe that the merger of St. Joseph and AMI will strengthen Creighton University's ability to function as one of the few Catholic academic health centers in the United States.

St. Joseph's clearly seeks to gain access to an expanded revenue base and to skilled management by this venture. But it is not obvious whether the sale of the hospital, rather than a lease or an affiliation arrangement, will best serve Creighton's needs. Nor are the specific controls and safeguards for the hospital's academic and social missions yet apparent. Rev. Morrison's hope for the continued "catholicity" of the hospital raises additional issues. What will be the extent of the control maintained? Will procedures considered wrong or ethically ambiguous by Catholic standards ever be performed under some circumstances? What concrete resources will the old, and the new, owners of the hospital have if conflicts arise?

Finally, in a new ownership situation like that of St. Joseph's, the academic partner seems particularly vulnerable to a pullout by the for-profit purchaser. What will happen should AMI choose at some future time either to sell out or close down the hospital? Such a decision, even for a flagship institution, could be based on factors separate from the specific profitability of St. Joseph's. It should be remembered that Humana for example, was principally in the nursing home business until it decided in 1972 to concentrate on hospitals and sell the more than 50 nursing homes it owned. A similar change-of-direction decision by AMI could leave Creighton with its teaching hospital in the hands of outsiders or else put a huge and sudden cash demand on the university, a demand it might well have trouble meeting at some future date.

C. Lease of a University Hospital by a For-Profit Hospital Chain

The two preceding cases illustrate the issues involved in direct ownership by a for-profit chain of a teaching and research facility – in one case, an independent facility (Humana Hospital-Audubon), and, in the other a pre-existing institution (Creighton). Humana's relationship with the University of Louisville (Health Services Information, 1984; Fact Sheet, 1983; Humana Hospital University, 1983) offers an example of a leasing arrangement between a chain and an existing academic medical center. Under the agreement, Humana is leasing the existing facilities of University Hospital – now called Humana Hospital University – for an initial four-year term at a rental of $6.5 million per year. The lease can then be renewed for another 36 years at a rental of $6 million per year. The corporation also is providing $4 million for necessary new equipment and will pay for the maintenance, upkeep, and operating expenses of the facilities that the company leases.

The agreement specifies several financial commitments to teaching and research. At the beginning of the fifth year, $4 million will be given to the University of Louisville School of Medicine to support education and research. An estimated $2.3 million will be provided by Humana – representing a major portion of the salaries and benefits for up to 174 residents – during the first educational year of the agreement. Future amounts will be renegotiated yearly. Space and facilities in the hospital will be provided free of charge for research programs. In addition, 20 percent of the Hospital's pretax profits will go to the University of Louisville.

Humana Hospital University is one of the clearest instances of a flagship situation. Louisville is the company's home base, and Humana may well be willing to take initial losses on the hospital for the sake of its local and national reputation. It is clear that the agreement supports the financial stability of the hospital's academic mission.

Questions persist, however. The dean of Louisville's medical school, has called the agreement's first year "relatively successful" but points out that "we find ourselves at times competing with the corporation's other hospitals for the resources and the programs and the patients" (Kmetz, 1984). While this kind of competition might be less of a problem in a community where a for-profit chain's activities were not so widespread as in Louisville, the marketplace interests of a chain might well interfere with the academic goals of a medical center. Where the balance of power in a lease arrangement lies with the for-profit partner, items subject to frequent renegotiation, like the residency support, might be likely losers. The relatively short-term renewal period of the lease – four years – may also be a potential threat to the academic mission of the hospital and will increase Humana's bargaining power especially in times of market recession. In four years, the for-profit company could take steps that markedly alter the patient mix of the leased university hospital, leaving a different institution, if options are not picked up or negotiations for continued operation fail.

D. Lease of a Psychiatric Hospital by a For-Profit Hospital Chain

Recent negotiations over the future of McLean Hospital, the well-known and highly respected psychiatric institution located in Belmont, Massachusetts, highlight a number of the options open to for-profit corporations desiring access to a flagship institution (Burr, 1984; Boston Globe, 1984). McLean is currently owned by the McLean Hospital Corporation, an affiliate of Massachusetts General Hospital Corporation. In the summer of 1983, the Hospital Corporation of America (HCA) made an offer to purchase the hospital while continuing to operate it as a teaching and research institution associated with Harvard Medical School (HMS). After a period of strongly argued and often highly public debate, the faculty of HMS rejected HCA's bid. The "overwhelmingly negative" faculty reaction to the proposal, as it was described in HMS Faculty Advisory Committee report on the issue, centered not on any specific characterization of HCA, but on a more general questioning of any purchase of the institution by a for-profit concern. The faculty rejection led to renewed negotiations between HCA and the McLean Hospital trustees and to a new HCA proposals to lease, rather than buy, McLean.

E. Ground Lease and Construction of a Psychiatric Hospital for a University Psychiatry Department by a For-Profit Company

In certain leasing arrangements, a for-profit company enters into ground lease arrangements with a university to build, equip, and operate a teaching/research facility. Such a project is underway in Tampa, where the University of Southern Florida (USF) has entered into an arrangement with the Forum Group of Indianapolis to build a 114-bed psychiatric teaching, research, and clinical facility for use by the university (Florida Board of Regents, 1984). A subsidiary of Forum Group, University Psychiatric Center, Inc. (UPC), is leasing 10 acres of land on the USF campus to erect the facility. The university is responsible for equipping, furnishing, and providing telephone service for the 10,0000 square feet of research space, and UPC is responsible for the rest of the facility. UPC will contract with USF to hire faculty and house staff for five percent of the previous year's net revenues. The for-profit partner will also pay the university 20 percent of its pre-tax profits in support of research and education at the new psychiatric hospital. At the end of the 40-year-lease period, the facility and land will return to the university.

Ideally, the university will receive a centralized teaching facility, along with sufficient research space (the agreement specifies 10,000 square feet) to further advance its teaching and research programs. UPC, in return, is gaining a high-quality for-profit psychiatric center and a close relationship with a major teaching institution that can offer Forum ready access to faculty expertise and technological advances for use at its other psychiatric hospitals.

The actual agreement entered into has a number of detailed provisions that, the parties hope, will serve as safeguards to the facility's social and academic mission. These include a board of directors representing both parties equally and formulae fixing the for-profit partner's contribution to teaching and research and indigent care at certain percentages of profits and/or revenue. Default on any term of the lease by either party is sufficient to terminate the lease.

Even with these provisions – or perhaps because of some of them – there may be a number of gaps in the protection afforded USF. The ease of termination – default on a single payment would suffice – enables Forum to withdraw quickly from the arrangement, forcing USF to consider a premature buy-back. This could occur if, due to changes in taxation or market conditions, Forum decided the hospital would yield little profit. USF, even if it could afford to buy Forum's interest, might be strained, at least in the short term, to provide the management expertise to run its own psychiatric teaching hospital.

The fixed-formula contributions also present potential drawbacks. Forum, in theory, could use company pricing policies to reduce pretax profits, thus limiting its annual payment to USF for teaching and research. In any event, pressures will exist on both USF and Forum to maximize patient census, thereby increasing revenue. This could conflict with the socially desirable goal of limiting hospitalization in cases where clinical efficacy is not obvious.

Finally, the USF Forum project is perhaps too small and involves too little public exposure to be a true flagship situation. It will thus have to justify itself, more than some other cooperative ventures, on straight business terms. Should the profitability of psychiatric practice decline, the teaching and research goals of the hospital might be jeopardized. To further complicate the issue, the Wall Street Journal, (1984) reported that Forum Group Inc. said it agreed in principle to sell its 14 hospitals of HCA for $194 million. Forum said it will now focus on its retirement communities for the "affluent elderly."

F. Contract Management

After leasing arrangements, management contracts form a logical next step in the spectrum of possible relationships between for-profit concerns and academic medical centers. Indeed, these contracts are increasingly widespread and raise some issues similar to those brought out earlier in this discussion. Since such contracts are generally limited in nature and much more easily dissolvable than ownership or lease arrangements, however, they present fewer long-term problems and, therefore, are not examined here.

G. Direct Grants

Financial support of education and research through direct grants from for-profit chains would appear to have the least impact on existing relationships. Yet, even in these cases, some significant changes should be expected. The for-profit chains, as they fund projects, have the potential to exercise an important influence over grant recipients and the subject matter of research.

There have been a number of such grants in recent years. AMI has contributed $150,000 to Harvard Medical School to support a new program designed to supplement students' technical training with general management skills (AMI Progress Report, 1984). AMI feels that the program, called "New Pathway to General Medical Education," parallels its own corporate emphasis on generalist executives. In April 1984, HCA announced a package of grants, totaling nearly one million dollars, to be made to Duke, Harvard, Washington, and Vanderbilt Universities and the Universities of Minnesota and Pennsylvania (Center for Health Studies, 1984). Among the topics studied will be the impact of HCA hospital acquisition, the nature and influence of HCA's corporate organization model, and comparisons of HCA hospital performance with hospitals run by not-for-profit systems.

The for-profit chains have also made direct grants for basic research. Humana contributed $1.4 million in 1983 to the University of Louisville School of Medicine to establish an institute to promote excellence in the research, diagnosis, and treatment of cardiovascular diseases. The new institute – separate from the Humana-Audubon Heart Institute – will include service, teaching, and research projects to strengthen the university's residency programs in cardiothoracic surgery at Humana Hospital University.

Another innovative program is HCA's incorporation of a non-profit charitable foundation to support health research and education. The company set aside two percent of its stock in 1982 as an initial endowment and hopes the fund's assets will exceed $100 million in the next five or six years. In addition to direct grants of its own, HCA will match, up to $500, charitable donations made to medical or dental schools by physicians or employees affiliated with company-owned facilities.

These grants are an intriguing first step toward programs of general aid to education and research. Yet, they are clearly not devoid of possible self-interest. Large-scale grants, made with appropriate fanfare, can serve some of the same purposes as the operation of a flagship institution. In addition, some of the funds and research produced by them can funnel back to benefit the for-profit chains. Humana's "Centers of Excellence" program specifically channels grants to physicians practicing in Humana-owned hospitals. The HCA grants to universities deal principally with organizational and administrative studies of HCA operations. The end products of the research may, in fact, differ only slightly from information produced by management consulting contracts that HCA might let out.

Even when basic research is involved, significant questions remain. How will a for-profit chain select grantees? Will they have peer review and, if so, under whose auspices? Will efforts be made to continuously analyze patterns of related interest, such as the links among Symbion, Dr. DeVries, and Humana? Here, too, as with the more direct, active forms of for-profit involvement, academic medical centers and researchers will have to exercise great caution.

All the relationships just discussed raise questions, but they also provide strong opportunities (Bowles, 1984). The necessary task is to discover what problems are inherent in ties between for-profit chains and the academic medical world and what problems can be solved through skillful negotiation. Already a battery of special arrangements–joint boards of directors, fixed-formula contributions, endowments, periodic reviews, and options to withdraw–have been tried. Others will no doubt soon be invented. If such tighter guarantees for the support and continuity of programs can be worked out, there will be a continued fruitful partnership between for-profit companies and academic medical centers. The key is to arrive at arrangements as airtight as possible before agreements are signed. Both university hospitals and for-profit hospital chains cannot assume that things will work out according to their best expectations. They must assume the worst to achieve the best.

Unless for-profit chains are legislatively impeded from participating in the academic health care, research, and education sectors, the relations described in this paper will grow. Institutions with primarily non-economic goals will have to learn to take advantage where they can and protect themselves where they must. Such a strategy may create de facto limits on the for-profit companies by limiting the profitability of certain relationships and by reducing the flexibility of companies to seek a maximum return on their investments. But that may prove better than making medical teaching and research potential hostages of the marketplace (Ginzberg, 1984; Cunningham, 1982; Relman, 1980). Research and education cannot be fully insulated from the business cycle, but inventiveness and some hard bargaining should enable them to benefit where they can.

REFERENCES

"AMI Discloses Plans to Buy Omaha Teaching Hospital." *FAH Review*, July/August 1984, 61.

Bowles, L. T. "The Influence of Medical Practice Competition on the Academic Medical Center's Educational Mission." *Journal of Medical Education*, 59(7):605–606, July 1984.

Burr, Francis H. (Chairman, Board of Trustees, McLean Hospital Corporation) Memo to Members of McLean Hospital Community, July 20, 1984.

Clark, M., Raine, G., and Ablow, K. "A Surgical Star Jumps Ship." *Newsweek*, August 13, 1984, p. 65.

Cunningham, R. "Changing Philosophies in Medical Care and the Rise of the Investor-Owned Hospital." *The New England Journal of Medicine*, 307(13):817–819, September 23, 1982.

"Forum to Sell Assets to Hospital Corp. for $194 Million." *The Wall Street Journal*, October 1, 1984, p. 13.

Ginzberg, E. "The Monetarization of Medical Care." *The New England Journal of Medicine*, 310(18):1162–1165, May 3, 1984.

"HCA's Committment to Medical Education and Research." Nashville: The Center for Health Studies, Hospital Corporation of America, June 15, 1984.

"Humana Focus: Technology." *The New York Times*, August 14, 1984, p. D1.

"Humana Hospital University: Six-Month Operations Report (*Fact Sheet*). Louisville: Humana Hospital University, December 8, 1983.

"Humana Hospital University: A Unique Health-Care Partnership." Louisville: Humana Hospital University, September 1983.

"Humana Takeover Reported Successful." *Health Services Information*, June 4, 1984 pp. 2–3.

Kmetz, Donald. "Investor-Owned Corporations and the Teaching Hospital." Unpublished paper presented at the Council of Teaching Hospitals meeting, May 1984.

Lease Agreement Between the Florida Board of Regents and University Psychiatric Center, Inc., March 23, 1984.

"Medical Grants." *AMI Progress Report*, January 1984, p. 7.

"Plan Under Way to Lease McLean." *The Boston Globe*, July 1, 1984, p. 37.

Relman, A. "The New Medical-Industrial Complex." *The New England Journal of Medicine*, 303(17):963–970, October 23, 1980.

"Surgeon's Move Highlights Controversial Trends." *The New York Times*, August 7, 1984, p. C3.

"Utah Surgeon Moving Heart Implant Program to Kentucky." *The New York Times*, August 1, 1984, p. A19.

Ruth S. Hanft, M.A.
Consultant in Health Policy Research, Washington, D.C.

The Implications for Teaching and Research

There is continued heated debate on the implications of the involvement of investor-owned firms in the health industry, the hospital sector, and teaching hospitals (Relman, 1980, 1983; Ginzberg, 1984; Sloan and Vraciu, 1983; Cunningham, 1983). Physician- and investor-owned hospitals have been the sites of education programs in osteopathy and psychiatry for some time. Although there are differences in the type, size, scope, and organization of allopathic and osteopathic training programs, as well as psychiatric and other medical and surgical residency programs, there are no empirical data to predict effects of the extension of this trend to all of allopathic medicine. There is, however, considerable rhetoric.

Opponents of the entry of investor-owned firms into teaching hospitals fear the end of medical education as we know it, particularly in terms of the loss of faculty and medical school control over education programs, the loss of autonomy of faculty, an emphasis on dollars rather than on education or care, a skew in the patient mix based on payment status, and a decline in clinical research activity. Proponents see greater efficiency and cost-effectiveness in the education process, improved quality of education and care with closer supervision of house staff, removal of a sometimes costly burden from universities, new revenue for universities and medical schools, and training that is more responsive to current and future community practice and to patient needs and satisfaction.

This is all conjecture. Time is needed to collect sufficient data to assess effects. When data are available, there will probably be validation of some of the fears and validation of some of the claims of improvement.

The issue of multi-organizational systems versus single institutional models generally is not raised as part of a discussion of for-profit/not-for-profit operation of teaching hospitals. Yet, it may have a more profound impact on hospital operations than ownership. The not-for-profits and the investor-owned hospitals may respond similarly to external forces (Heyssel, 1981).

Since there are no objective data and so few examples of for-profit ownership or lease of teaching hospitals, this paper attempts to set the context for discussion and raise the issues that should be studied.

SOME MYTHS AND REALITIES

The health care field, perhaps more than any other field, has a plethora of interests that tend to foster general ideological perceptions often based on myths rather than realities. Some of these myths are germane to assessing whether for-profit/not-for-profit status makes a difference.

Myth 1: Teaching hospitals place their highest priority on education programs.

Teaching hospitals are part of a very diverse university and few generalizations apply to all of them (Worthington, 1981). Teaching hospitals have multiple missions that include patient care, the education of many types of students, and clinical research. Some, if they can afford to do so, give top priority to education, but the majority do not, and, over the past few years, the pressures to maintain financial viability have increased the attention given to the patient care mission and efficiency (Iglehart, 1982; Association of Academic Health Centers, 1983). Profit and loss is as much an issue for not-for-profit hospitals as it is for the investor-owned hospitals, although the ultimate distribution of these profits differs.

Myth 2: If teaching hospitals are sold or leased to for-profit companies, medical schools will lose control over the graduate medical education programs.

Only 62 teaching hospitals are university-owned, and it is only in these that there is a real possibility for total control of graduate medical education (GME) by the medical school. A number of large, high-quality graduate medical education programs have always been controlled by the hospital rather than the medical school. For example, Massachusetts General Hospital and Montefiore in New York, although closely affiliated with the Harvard and Albert Einstein Medical Schools, respectively, make the major decisions on their residency programs. At numerous community hospital teaching programs, the hospital plays the dominant role. In most principal teaching hospitals owned by universities, the clinical chairman has been dominant rather than the medical school. During the last five years, most medical schools have had to negotiate with hospital administration on the size and scope of education programs as one of the realities of cost containment (Iglehart, 1982; Association of Academic Health Centers, 1983; Smith and Stemmler, 1981).

Myth 3: If teaching hospitals become for-profit institutions, they no longer provide uncompensated care, the corollary being that all teaching hospitals currently provide uncompensated care (Association of Academic Health Centers, 1982, 1983; Feder and Hadley, 1983).

Although teaching hospitals provide a disproportionate amount of uncompensated care compared with nonteaching hospitals, not all teaching hospitals provide large amounts of uncompensated care. Most of those that do are county- or state-owned university hospitals, inner-city teaching hospitals with historic commitments to serve the total population of the community, or hospitals that must based on Hill-Burton requirements. There have been a number of reports of restrictions imposed on uncompensated care by teaching hospitals that heretofore had open door policies (Association of Academic Health Centers, 1982 and 1983).

Myth 4: For-profit teaching hospitals will have a less-rich case mix of patients and less severely ill patients. Hence, students will not have an appropriate clinical base.

Teaching hospitals have a richer case mix than nonteaching hospitals and also a wider range of case mixes (Johns Hopkins Center for Hospital Finance and Management, 1984). There is no current evidence that for-profit teaching hospitals will have a different case mix distribution than most not-for-profit teaching hospitals. Furthermore, if a for-profit teaching hospital serves as a referral center for its own vertical system or for a region, or if the medical school has access to state-of-the-art care in another hospital in the corporation, the case mix may become far more complex and desirable from an education perspective.

Myth 5: For-profit hospitals will not support unfunded clinical research.

Not all teaching hospitals support unfunded clinical research. Few not-for-profit hospitals can continue to support unfunded clinical research unless they are subsidized by the state or cross-subsidized by profit-making services. The changes in reimbursement, the development of preferred provider organizations (PPOs), and increased health maintenance organization (HMO) activity may have more impact on the quantity of unfunded clinical research than ownership or lease for hospitals (Bergen and Roth, 1984). In fact, Humana, Inc., is directly investing in clinical research by funding a cardiovascular research Center of Excellence.

Myth 6: The medical schools will lose a source of support from patient care revenues.

There is no evidence that medical schools will lose revenue. A number of medical schools are experiencing a decline in hospital payments for faculty, even from university-owned hospitals. If the patient base of a hospital erodes through inability to compete, whether the hospital is investor-owned or not-for-profit, practice plan revenues will be affected. If, as anticipated by some observers, investor-owned hospitals stimulate increased faculty productivity, medical school revenues may rise rather than fall. The trend in practice plan revenues continues to show an increase (*Journal of the American Medical Association*, 1984).

TEACHING HOSPITAL CONTEXT

Of the approximately 1,500 teaching hospitals in the United States, the majority have five or fewer residency programs (Smith and Stemmler, 1984). Some of these hospitals are almost indistinguishable from nonteaching community hospitals. The most recent Accreditation Committee on Graduate Medical Education Directory of Residency Training Programs reports that there were more than 72,000 residents in approved teaching programs in September 1983. One hundred non-federal hospitals that were members of the Council of Teaching Hospitals trained 46 percent of the house staff (Smith and Stemmler, 1984). The Veterans Administration trained another 12 percent. Almost 60 percent of residents are trained by a small proportion of teaching hospitals. In addition, more than half of the residency training takes place in eight states: New York, California, Pennsylvania, Texas, Illinois, Ohio, Massachusetts, and Michigan. There are approximately 150–175 institutions that I would call major teaching hospitals. These hospitals (except for children's hospitals) have programs in most fields and more than 100 house staff based at the hospital. The Association of American Medical Colleges gives a more conservative estimate of 110–115 hospitals in this category.

Even among these 150–175 institutions, there are major differences in ownership, relationship to medical schools, uncompensated care, case mix, and financial viability. Of these hospitals, about 60 are owned outright by universities; some are public and receive appropriations from their state legislatures (Council of Teaching Hospitals, 1984); and others are private, receiving no special treatment from the state. Even among state or university-owned hospitals, there are major differences in size and responsibility. The Medical College of Virginia, for example, serves as a major tertiary care center for a large region of Virginia and also has a very large proportion of indigent patients. The University of California at Los Angeles (UCLA) Hospital, also a tertiary care center, serves a much lower proportion of indigent patients because of the extensive county hospital system and UCLA's responsibility for patient care services in a county hospital. UCLA also has several tertiary care competitors in the area. Size of university hospitals varies from around 300 beds to 1,000 beds. Like public university hospitals, private university hospitals show considerable differences in size, uncompensated care, and case mix.

Most medical schools do not own their hospitals. A number of universities have always relied on independent teaching hospitals to provide clinical education. Most notable perhaps are the Harvard-Massachusetts General/Brigham/Beth Israel arrangements and the University of Southern Calfornia-Los Angeles County relationship.

A number of universities rely heavily on county and municipal hospitals to provide clinical training for their students even when the university owns its hospital. The university hospital, in effect, is the "private" hospital, and the county hospital provides most of the uncompensated care. Examples of universities with dependence on county or municipal hospitals are Emory and Tulane.

The role of the Veterans Administration (VA) hospitals cannot be underestimated. Without these, a number of medical schools, even those that own their hospitals, would not have sufficient clinical base for training. In addition, the Veterans Administration funded the development and expansion of medical schools in the 1970s to enhance the staffing and quality of care in VA hospitals. Wright State, East Tennessee, and Marshall are relatively new medical schools started with the assistance of VA funding.

Finally, most of the medical schools or campus branches of an existing school that began operating within the last two decades were designed as community-based schools with clinical training provided in pre-existing community and/or VA hospitals. Examples include the University of Kansas at Wichita and the Eastern Virginia Medical Authority.

In addition to differences in ownership, size, and relation to universities, there are major differences in the role of the medical school plays in decisions about control of education programs and size of house staff. Control of education programs within university-owned hospitals usually rests with department chairmen, but this is rapidly changing as deans, vice chancellors, and hospital administrators assume more authority (Association of Academic Health Centers, 1982 and 1983). At some major teaching hospitals, there are both integrated and non-integrated residency programs, although the latter have declined. The medical school may play a minor role in size or selection of house staff or supervision of the program even when the clinical chairman at the hospital is on the faculty of the medical school. Prior to the 1960s, medical schools were largely responsible for undergraduate medical students and some schools were primarily basic science schools with the hospitals the locus of graduate medical education and clinical clerkships.

EXTERNAL ENVIRONMENT

Until recent changes in reimbursement, support for graduate medical education, undergraduate clinical education and unfunded clinical research was not a problem (except in cases where a teaching hospital provided large amounts of uncompensated care). These costs simply were passed on to the care payers either directly or indirectly through cost shifting. There was little reason for university-owned hospitals of any sort, to consider sale or lease to an investor-owned chain.

Although the direct and indirect costs of graduate medical education are still passed through under Medicare and most third-party payers, a number of other recent phenomena are influencing attitudes toward ownership and are changing the behavior of the not-for-profit sector.

Diagnosis-related groups (DRGs) placed incentives on the use of fewer services per diagnosis, greater efficiency of management, and shorter hospital stays. There is still a paucity of data on the costs of graduate medical education and whether and in what proportion increased costs are a function of education, case mix, and inefficiency (Hanft, 1982; Horn, 1983). The closer their ties to a medical school, the more hospitals have responded to pressures from the schools regarding the number of staff, the credentials of nurses, and the autonomy of faculty and staff requests for equipment and the like. How much these factors have influenced costs is not known (Bergen and Roth, 1984).

Preferred provider organizations (PPOs), a relatively new development, and the rapid growth of HMOs are placing additional pressures on teaching hospitals by forcing them to compete on a price basis (Association of Academic Health Centers, 1982 and 1983). Admissions and lengths of stay are declining throughout the country, thereby affecting the hospital base for clinical training.

Federal support through direct grants continues to decline, and support of research declined in constant dollars until fiscal year 1984 (Hanft and Fishman, 1984). State appropriations for health professions education have declined as a proportion of total state expenditures due to pressures to support other social programs.

A number of universities are concerned about the potential drain of the university hospital on the university as a whole. Some universities have subsidized their hospitals from endowments or have absorbed hospital losses by cutting other important programs. Governance problems and tradition inhibit the ability of some hospitals, particularly state and university-owned hospitals, to respond to change. Constraints exist in civil service or university personnel and procurement systems, and diffusion of decision making reduces flexibility to respond rapidly to change (Hanft, 1983; Ebert, et. al., 1983; Munson, 1982). It may be easier to sell or lease than to change governance.

Not-for-profit teaching hospitals have begun to respond to change by establishing for-profit subsidiaries; changing governance, management style, and admissions policies; and reducing the autonomy of the education community within their walls. Some teaching hospitals have now become part of multi-hospital organizations; of course, these new relationships will affect decisions on teaching programs. State university hospitals have also begun to make changes in governance. Recently, hospitals of the Universities of Maryland, Washington, and West Virginia have changed their governance structure, making themselves more independent of the state and university.

Venture capital, particularly for state hospitals and inner city hospitals, is increasingly difficult to obtain; yet, for these hospitals to remain state-of-the-art institutions, capital must be available.

Until recently, the issue of sale or lease of university and principal hospitals to investor-owned hospitals simply was not considered. The Hospital Corporation of America, until the acquisition of Wesley Hospital in Wichita, Kansas, had been unsuccessful in its attempts to purchase or assume total responsibility for a teaching hospital. With the growing fiscal constraints, residency review requirements, and a potential decline in the number of medical students, it is virtually impossible today for a nonteaching hospital to become a major teaching hospital *de novo*. Within the last two years, the University of Louisville's and Creighton University's teaching hospitals were respectively leased and sold to investor-owned corporations.

POSSIBLE MOTIVATIONS TO CHANGE FROM NONTEACHING TO TEACHING STATUS OR TO ACQUIRE A TEACHING HOSPITAL

As long as teaching costs can be passed through, absorbed by state funding or made sufficiently reasonable to justify a trade-off in service and quality, motives for acquiring a teaching hospital could include competition, quality of care throughout the system, and perceived ability to maintain or enhance profit and prestige.

A vertical system or a PPO or HMO arrangement must be able to provide or contract for a full range of services, including tertiary care. Services that require backup, 24-hour staffing, and state-of-the-art equipment (e.g., shock trauma, transplant surgery, experimental chemotherapy) are generally found only in teaching hospitals. The formation of multi-hospital, not-for-profit systems that include teaching hospitals gives a competitive edge to not-for-profit systems unless investor-owned systems acquire or contract with teaching institutions.

Physicians are likely to try to locate in the area where they completed their residency training. They tend to refer to the hospitals where they were trained and to the specialists who trained them. Clearly, it behooves a hospital to have a base of loyal referring physicians or a pool of physicians who will consider employment with the hospital or hospital-sponsored services.

Teaching hospitals, particularly major teaching hospitals, have early access to new technology often subsidized by manufacturers or the National Institutes of Health (NIH), giving them a competitive edge over other hospitals. Diffusion of new technology starts with teaching hospitals that train the physicians in use of these technologies. Physicians then bring this knowledge to community hospitals. Many observers of academic health centers have noted that the teaching hospitals and their faculty train their future competitors.

American corporations in other fields have made community contributions to education and research and other societal goods as part of the concept of "corporate conscience," even when there is a loss of profit. These activities are undertaken to gain prestige and the respect of the community and because of a genuine interest in community affairs. Teaching hospitals, particularly principal teaching hospitals of universities, are widely regarded as prestigious national or regional institutions.

ISSUES FOR EVALUATING THE EFFECTIVE FOR-PROFIT OPERATION OF TEACHING HOSPITALS

There are four criteria on which society should evaluate the effects of the entry of investor-owned hospitals into the education arena: size and quality of education programs, financing of medical and graduate medical education, scope and quantity of clinical research, and access to care.

Size and Quality of the Program

The size of residency programs in some institutions is declining. Therefore, analysis of change must include comparison of regional and national trends and rates of change among all programs. Termination of a program by a hospital would be an indicator, depending on who initiated the action and why. Discontinuation of certain types of services by the hospital or transfer of services within the multi-hospital system or to another nonteaching site can also affect the residency programs. Again, analysis of the rationale for change is needed before conclusions can be drawn.

Qualitative issues can objectively be measured only to a degree. Considerable reliance could be placed on accreditation reviews by residency review committees and accreditation visits of the Liaison Committee for Medical Education. Other bases include scores on standardized national board and specialty certification exams for students; recruitment and retention of outstanding faculty; shifts of faculty among affiliations, changes in the use of volunteer and part-time faculty; changes in the levels of supervision of house staff, and house staff autonomy in admissions and in ordering services.

House staff autonomy remains a controversial issue. At the Mayo Clinic – a highly regarded education program – faculty supervision of house staff is strict. In other well-regarded programs, supervision is less intense or is graduated by year of residency. Because of the cost implications of autonomy under current Medicare reimbursement and price competition, however, the trend is to increase the level of supervision of house staff in all teaching hospitals.

Financing of Medical and Graduate Medical Education

Medical schools derive considerable revenues and indirect benefits from patient care activities that take place in hospitals and clinics. These revenues come from three sources: hospital payment for faculty supervision of house staff, payment of house staff salaries with house staff spending some time teaching medical students, and practice plan revenues.

Evaluation of trends in each of the streams of support is needed. My hypothesis is that over time there might be a reduction in revenues from the first two sources, due to more cost-effective management, and an increase in the third source, due to stronger emphasis on the importance of faculty activities in patient care and patient satisfaction. There may be potential for a new source of revenue if there is a development of profit-sharing agreements between hospitals and medical schools.

Scope and Quantity of Clinical Research

Major teaching hospitals traditionally have been the site of clinical research and clinical trials. Although most of the research is funded by NIH and other biomedical research grants, the hospital may provide space, staff time, supplies and equipment. But the factors noted previously in the section External Environment are affecting the ability of hospitals to continue these types of investments. It will be very difficult to evaluate whether changes occur because of changes in hospital ownership for two primary reasons: difficulty in separating the effects of competition and of changed reimbursement, and difficulty in measuring the prior and present levels of research (this has never been done). The only available evaluation tools are trends in research grant support for medical school clinical departments, direct grants to hospitals, and before-and-after studies of faculty activity.

Access to Care: Uncompensated and Indigent Care

Teaching hospitals vary widely in the amount of uncompensated care they provide. Changes in this can affect the clinical teaching case mix, thereby reducing or increasing exposure of students to different types of patients and to different types of diagnoses. For example, hypertension, diabetes, low-birthweight infants and certain forms of cancer occur more frequently among the non-white, low-income population. Changes in case mix can be measured by changes in volume, by diagnostic categories, and, as a proxy, by source of patient payment. Changes are now occurring in the not-for-profit sector, with public hospitals experiencing increases in uncompensated patients as not-for-profit voluntary hospitals limit their volume of uncompensated care (Hanft, 1982). The increased limitation on access nationally remains a serious public policy issue with consequences for the scope and quality of care and education.

REFERENCES

Arthur Young & Co. *Financing of Medical Education*, forthcoming.

Association of Academic Health Centers. *Impact of Changes in Federal Policy on Academic Health Centers*. Washington, D.C., October 1982.

Association of Academic Health Centers. *Impact of Changes in Federal Policy on Academic Health Centers Academic Health Centers Revisited*. Washington, D.C., July 1983.

Bergen, Stanley M. and Roth, Amy. "Prospective Payment and the University Hospital." *The New England Journal of Medicine*, 310(5):316–318, February 2, 1984.

Bromberg, Michael. "The Medical-Industrial Complex: Our National Defense." *The New England Journal of Medicine*, 309(21):1314, November 24, 1983.

Council of Teaching Hospitals. Unpublished data from annual survey of university-owned teaching hospitals: financial and general operating data. Washington, D.C.: Association of American Medical Colleges, 1984.

Cunningham, Robert Jr. "Entrepeneuralism in Medicine." *The New England Journal of Medicine*, 309(21):1313, November 24, 1983.

Ebert, Robert H. and Brown, Sarah S. "Academic Health Centers." *The New England Journal of Medicine*, 308(20):1200–1208, May 19, 1983.

"Eighty-Fourth Annual Report on Medical Education in the United States, 1983–84." *The Journal of the American Medical Association*, 255(12):1241–1253, September 28, 1984.

Feder, Judith and Hadley, Jack. "Hospital Care to the Poor in 1980." Urban Institute Working Paper 3179-04, August 1983.

Ginzberg, Eli. "The Monetarization of Medical Care." *The New England Journal of Medicine*, 310(18):1162–1165, May 3, 1984.

Hanft, Ruth S. "The Impact of Changes in Federal Policy on Academic Health Centers." *Health Affairs*, l(4):70–82, Fall 1982.

Hanft, Ruth S. and Fishman, Linda E. "The Reagan FY 1985 Budget and Medicare, Medicaid and Health Programs." *Federal Budget Report*, The Reagan 1985 Budget Series, March 1984.

Heyssel, Robert. "Commercial Stress and The Academic Medical Center." Presented at the Annual Meeting of the Association of American Medical Colleges, Washington, D.C., November 3, 1981.

Horn, Susan D. "Does Severity of Illness Make a Difference in Prospective Payment." *Health Care Financial Management*. 13(5):49–53, May 1983.

Iglehart, John K. "Moment of Truth for the Teaching Hospitals." *The New England Journal of Medicine*, 307(2):132–136, July 8, 1982.

Munson, F. C. "Management and Governance of University Hospitals." Unpublished paper delivered at the Association of Academic Health Centers Fall Meeting, October 2, 1982.

Relman, Arnold S. "The New Medical-Industrial Complex." *The New England Journal of Medicine*, 303(17):963–970, October 23, 1980.

Relman, Arnold S. "Investor-Owned Hospitals and Health Care Costs." *The New England Journal of Medicine*, 309(6):370–372, August ll, 1983.

Sloan, Frank A. and Vraciu, R. A. "Investor-Owned and Not-for-Profit Hospitals: Addressing Some Issues." *Health Affairs*, 2(l):25–37, Fall 1983.

Smith, Thomas C. and Stemmler, Edward J. "Financing of Undergraduate and Graduate Medical Education." Testimony before the Subcommittee on Health, U.S. Senate Committee on Finance, October 1, 1984.

Worthington, Nancy L. "Measuring Hospitals' Educational Project: A Typology of the U.S. Teaching Hospitals." Prepared for the Annual Meeting of the American Public Health Association, Los Angeles, California, November 3, 1981.

Discussion – Teaching and Research

Mr. Melvin Glasser, *Director, Health Security Action Council*: In the presentations, we have heard assurances from the medical school administrators and representatatives of the prospective purchasers that there is mutual trust and integrity . . . that whatever agreement may be worked out between the parties will doubtless be carried out fully in letter and in spirit. I have no basis for questioning this.

I know, however, that the health care field is currently in a great state of flux. Mergers, the organization of new corporations, new stock offerings are very much under discussion. I know, too, that major corporations, not now in the health field, are actively seeking new areas for investment of their burgeoning assets – companies like the R. J. Reynolds Corporation, MGM, or Mobil.

Has consideration been given to what might occur if sometime after the sale of this hospital, the investor owner were to sell out or be bought out by a company like those named – without background or previous involvement with the commitments made to this hospital? What are the implications for the future of the hospital – for the earlier good faith promises made?

Further, I wonder if the university and the medical school staffs have considered how they might feel if a year or two after sale their stationery might be changed to read "George Washington University Medical School – a subsidiary of the R. J. Reynolds Tobacco Company."

Dr. Ronald Kaufman, *Moderator, Vice President for Medical Affairs, The George Washington University*: In the experience of any of the three speakers has there been discussions of the implications for any proposed marriage, or other arrangement, in the event that companies like R. J. Reynolds, MGM, or Mobil were to buy out one of these for-profit corporations.

I think these three, because they are indeed acquisition minded, have no problems with moving outside the areas where they now function and have the money to acquire many of the hospital corporations.

Dr. Richard Egdahl, *Director, Boston University Medical Center and the Center for Industry and Health Care*: I think it is highly likely that this type of thing will occur as time goes on. The predictions are that in 20 or 30 years we may have ten or 15 very, very large companies. The biggest corporations are doing this. I am less clear as to what the implications will be. Those companies have problems, but they are highly ethical in terms of the way they operate, make a profit, and continue to satisfy the public in some way, or they do not survive.

So I sense the impact of your question and the problems that they contain. I am not sure, though, that the very size of the HCA at this point in time is not a great advantage in its capital generation. And one could perhaps think of some advantages from that, if it did not become a totally dominant form of profitability.

Ms. Ruth Hanft, *Consultant in Health Policy Research, Washington, D.C.*: Yes, I think there is an overriding consideration that we cannot answer yet that may be the clue to that, and that is what happens to hospital financial viability in terms of operating cost as PPOs and HMOs negotiate discounts and the competition stiffens as the patients move out of the hospital.

One of those three corporations might not find it a good investment for their stockholders five years down the pike. And I just do not think we know yet what the effects of these changes to universities are going to have.

I think it is entirely possible that some of the investor-owned hospital companies now, and some of them are diversifying like Humana, may actually reduce their investment in the hospital field if the reimbursement warrants it.

Mr. Samuel Mitchell, *Director of Research, Federation of American Hospitals*: My question is, to what extent is this issue worth worrying about now given that academic medical centers need capital and investor-owned hospitals have capital? Besides, academic medical centers are under no compulsion to sell; they can and do stipulate the terms under which they will let themselves be purchased.

Mr. Philip S. Birnbaum, *Dean for Administrative Affairs, The George Washington University*: We speculate that that already has a significant effect on their owning hospitals. I agree with Ruth: I think it is likely that some of the hospital-based chains will start reducing their interests in hospitals. For us it was a question of what other options there were, and what sort of safeguards can be included in relationships; safeguards that are enforceable.

Dr. Cecil Sheps, *Taylor Grandy Distinguished Professor of Social Medicine, The University of North Carolina at Chapel Hill*: One of the jobs I have held is that of General Director of one of the Harvard teaching hospitals, the Beth Israel in Boston. And I would suggest that a key element in Birnbaum's presentation is that matter of the level-one decision. They would be made by the medical center within the constraints set by AMI after consultation with the medical center. Let's examine that in terms of ultimate authority. The ultimate authority clearly is AMI.

I suggest to you that there is a difference, a crucial difference, between that kind of discussion and the kinds of discussions that my board and I in Boston used to have with the dean of the medical school. When the Harvard Medical School wanted us to do certain things because the School needed it, we did our best to get it done. We made those decisions not on the basis of whether we could make money, but whether in the overall scheme of things in the immediate sense or in the course of time, it would be sensible for us to provide that particular service.

The ultimate controlling factor was of course money but, subsidiary and affecting that continuously, was consideration of the nature of our institution and its social commitment, not only to the community of Boston but to Harvard Medical School. And I suggest to you that this represents a crucial difference in contrast to what is projected here today.

Ms. Ruth Hanft: I am not convinced that a hospital corporation has any less commitment, if they undertake what they consider a social obligation, than the Beth Israel. I do not think the world is as it was ten, 15, or 20 years ago. And I am watching university hospitals and not-for-profit teaching hospitals behaving very much like businesses. And I just think there has been a narrowing of differences. I do not think unless you were told that you would know that the ownership of certain institutions –

Dr. Cecil Sheps: I simply suggest that the reason for being has some effect, countered by various others. I am simply stressing attention to the institution's reason for being, that's all.

Mr. Melvin Glasser: I point out we have a window in time for this "profit for health" potential move. The window gives us a chance to build in to the flagship situations we are largely talking about today, certain arrangements that could benefit selling owner. There are examples now occurring where investor purchasers as well as current owners are setting up endowment funds to provide for continuing payments for uncompensated care.

I think that if you simply join in and then drift along and then get sold off when you prove to be a bad deal and do not have any reserves, that's not only stupid, it's improvident. But I think there are some chances now for some negotiations that help your unfunded poor, help your teaching obligations, and also benefit the for-profit change. And I think that that is what we have to look for in the negotiating process.

Ms. Helen Darling, *Director, Human Resources Studies, Government Research Corporation*: I do not know what number we are up to, but I would hope that the idea that research is not controlled by the nonprofit governmental world would be added to our list of myths. It may not be happening at NIH, but as a principal investigator a number of years ago for the Social Security Administration, I have had study results held up because they were not consistent with what the people wanted to have set for the world. I am not the only one; it happens all the time. This is not to suggest that it is not important that that be protected wherever we can, but it is not one-sided.

My question is, what does AMI or any one of the organizations that gets into this kind of thing really get out of it? I think Ruth put her finger on it a few minutes ago in her reaction about investors. A very large proportion of the investment on health care in this country is held by large pension funds that are mounted by institutional investors who spend a lot of time moving enormous chunks of money around. I can imagine that an awful lot of thought has gone into it by AMI or others in similar sorts of arrangements, so what they are going to get out of it is two-pronged in terms of the world to which they must be answerable.

Dr. John H. Moxley III, *Senior Vice President, American Medical International, Inc.*: I cannot improve really upon what Ruth said. I can add that, as we look to the future, we see larger and larger systems of care, direct purchasers of care having much greater influence, demanding more comprehensiveness all the way from home health care to the most tertiary levels of care. Therefore, there is a rationale for saying that if you are going to be in the future as it is now seen, one is going to have to broaden to that level.

Further, there is more to a relationship than can be developed as part of the original affiliation. A series of agreements between faculty members and the system in terms of continuing education, access to the data bases, etc., could be developed. There should be no question that these organizations, these companies could not be doing it if there was not a rationale, that there could be a reasonable return upon the investment.

Clearly, if a study were done at George Washington or XYZ University and the results were that the university teaching hospital was in a loss situation and nothing could be done to turn that loss situation around, there would be a very serious and inhibiting effect upon further discussion.

There is, I think, a commitment to what the academic centers stand for on the part of the management. I can speak personally for AMI. American health care is, no matter how much we scream about it, the best in the world. When I was in the Defense Department, I traveled all over the world, and I never went to a country that would not do most anything to get our system. The reason is that the system is scientifically based and by and large that science springs from academic centers. There is a thought, a conviction, that that ought to be preserved along with everything else, not in isolation, it makes sense, therefore, to move in the direction of mutually beneficial relationships.

Clearly, as everybody has indicated thus far this morning, time will tell. There are no measurements out there now. This is a new situation, and it will have to be monitored.

Dr. Jack Meyer, *Director, Center for Health Policy Research, American Enterprise Institute*: I would like to suggest that there is a problem of a red herring in this issue of the role for-profits in the hospital sector and health care generally. In fact, Warren, I think I would suggest a slight modification in the title of the conference from the implications of the for-profit hospital in health care, which I think at this point are unknown and fairly limited, to the implications of bringing the business mentality to health care.

And I would like to second Ruth's point, both the one that she made recently and in her paper, that it is really a certain behavior which we can find examples of in all the sectors of health care that is of interest. And what is of concern is that as we adopt more of a business mentality in health care, a lot more people are going to fall out of the bottom end of the market. We are going to have a greater need for safety valves that we do not now have.

Now, the answer to that problem is not a knee-jerk reaction against profitability, any more than it would be a reaction against chaining, which is by no means the exclusive problem of the for-profit world, or against management reforms. The answer is to allow those kind of reforms to play themselves out, with safeguards, but to compensate those that cannot play in that world.

I feel that issues such as remoteness of leadership (a management problem) and fear of people with high-risk conditions are not exclusive to the for-profit sector, and should be addressed in broader terms.

That leads me to my comment on Ruth's observation and her very honest statement about merit goods. I think that health care can be thought of as a merit good, like nutrition and housing. That does not lead me to want to dictate the ownership form or the markets outcome. Rather, it leads me to say that the government ought to compensate for the outcome of the market, if it is unhappy with the outcome, and allow market forces to play out.

I think that the real issue is how to fund indigent care and medical education through direct subsidies without interfering with the management economies that are unfolding.

Also, I think that instead of pondering over the proper form of ownership, we should be devising tax collection and redistribution schemes to provide these direct subsidies. If indigent care is unevenly distributed across the hospital sector by ownership, there are ways of dealing with that without changing the distribution by taxing and redistributing the funds. I just think we need to have an idea of who the real culprit is out there.

Finally, let me comment on the issue that Dick raised, which I think is a very important one, about the possible sullying of the researcher and interference with the independence of the researcher.

Very frankly, I think those conflicts of interest can potentially occur in all studies, not just in the for-profit world.

Dr. Gary Filerman, *President, Association of University Programs in Health Administration*: I'd like to make two comments. First, there was an interesting link between the Egdahl flagship concept and the Birnbaum description of the model that is involved in the AMI discussion. That was revealed in Birnbaum's comment about the possible relationship between this particular project and its networking potential with other activities in the region under the same corporate umbrella.

One of the things a flagship does is get them into the ocean. It's very important that in looking at specific academic health centers, we do not view them independently from the service community of which they are a part.

Although there may be a tendency to evaluate a particular unit (such as this hospital or any other teaching hospital) in terms of profitability of that particular enterprise it might make more sense to look at the entry that it provides to the total service area and surrounding facilities.

Some of the areas around this town are highly competitive, or at least potentially highly competitive for entry. I would suggest that anybody who is in an academic health center has dealt themselves a loaded deck in terms of access to the surrounding counties when the issues arise about access to and control of future health care facilities in those areas.

The second point I want to make is directed to the education area. The topic is not medical education, it is education. We are reflecting a bias in our discussion, a preoccupation with medical education, which is of some concern to me, since other health sciences educations are at stake in this process, as well.

The DRG impact on access to clinical facilities for health sciences education broadly defined is an issue that we are going to have to deal with. There are numerous community education programs which are university and college based. We are not dealing with 120 academic health centers, we are dealing with every college and university that has a nursing program, physical therapy program, and other programs that have increasing dependence on the hospital down the street for clinical access.

All of those programs are potentially in real trouble. The cost issues on their relations with the hospital down the street are changing rapidly. DRGs are part of it, proprietary or profits are another part of it, and they are going to raise some real questions about the viability of a lot of these programs in terms of their clinical needs.

Dr. Dennis O'Leary, *Dean for Clinical Affairs, The George Washington University School of Medicine and Health Sciences*: I would like to move back to the graduate medical education issue but not divorce myself entirely from the educational issue.

I think that this environment that we are living in now creates an opportunity to re-evaluate the hospital as a place where medical education or education in health sciences goes on. Let's not kid ourselves, the reason why graduate medical education has been focused very heavily on in the hospital is because that is where the funding for it has come from. That does not mean that we have not created appropriate rationales which we believe, to support this hospital-focused educational effort.

I am an internist, and my discipline has taken the basic philosophy that you have to train internists on really tough cases in the hospital. The corollary is that any idiot can learn how to take care of patients who are on the hoof. Now, point in fact, that's not true, and we have a certain number of idiots out there who do not know how to take care of ambulatory patients at all. What we do have is a lot of technicians who know the modalities of technological medicine and who, incidently, do not refer cases back to the tertiary academic medical centers but rather refer their cases to other tertiary care community hospitals throughout the Washington area.

I think that the threats that are posed to the funding of graduate medical education and to many of our other educational programs provide us with an opportunity to look at what we should be doing and how this should be funded for the future. One of the things that is in the hearts of our faculty in looking at a potential relationship with AMI or anyone else is what a wonderful opportunity to assure some financial stability for the funding of our house staff, if appropriate. So if this relationship moves forward, I hope that AMI and GW will look at this whole issue very carefully and, if dollars are an incentive, reshape the programs if possible.

If we create a vertical care system, perhaps a broad consideration should be exploring opportunities for educating our students and house staff in those settings which are most relevant to their future professional careers.

Mr. Samuel Mitchell: I think any serious observer would agree with Dr. Egdahl's points that there are going to be problems in academic medical center affiliations. Those problems are not going to go away, and they have to be dealt with on a case-by-case contract-by-contract basis. But I think the point that there are going to be problems has to be put in context.

Academic medical centers need capital, and there are really only three ways they can get capital. One is through affiliations with people with capital. Two, through increasing prices, and that's not doable in today's world. And three is government.

If you distribute money to academic medical centers through the tax system or through grants, my guess is that you are going to have a wide distribution of financing instead of a concentration in the quality institutions. If you finance incremental capital through affiliations with investor-owned hospitals, I think you will see less capital going to the second, third and fourth rank teaching hospitals, and an increase in the share of capital going to the first, the top-level academic medical centers.

Ms. Ruth Hanft: What I am worried about – and I did not bring this out in my statement – is that I am just as concerned as Jack about growing needs in the uncompensated care area. What will happen is that we are going to starve to death the L.A. County hospitals, the Bellevues. As the patients move out of the not-for-profit sector, as they get dumped – which is happening all over the country – as those publics cannot maintain capital plant, we are going to have an increasingly dual care system. Additionally, we are going to have medical schools like USC, whose students will only work in lack-of-state-of-the-art facilities because the capital is not there. Patients will not have access to the state of the art, and that's my worry. It has nothing to do with the for-profits and not-for-profits, it has to do with what is happening to uncompensated care and what is happening to the public hospitals in this country.

Dr. Ronald P. Kaufman: I thought that Dr. O'Leary was going to suggest that perhaps we have too many students and house staff being trained in our university hospitals rather than other settings.

I think we are going to note a trend away from a high percent of medical school training in the tertiary care hospital setting. I totally agree with Gary Filerman when he said he was very concerned about the other health professional schools with hundreds of field locations, many in hospitals immediately affected by waivers or DRGS.

Finally, I am for a free enterprise system for both nonprofits and for-profits. My only warning is that one must constantly focus on one's fundamental mission.

Mr. Philip Birnbaum: Let me underline that a major result of our study is the need for safeguards, the reality of those safeguards, and the conservation of resources to back up the safeguards. Underlying all of our concerns is the question that was just raised: What are the options open to the academic health centers in teaching hospitals?

Dr. Cecil Sheps: Mr. Birnbaum, in quickly reviewing the sources of capital, did not mention revenue bonds. I am wondering why that is and whether that does not remain as a possible source. What is the nature of the capital problem at GW in terms of source? Why was the revenue bond option discarded if it was considered?

Mr. Philip Birnbaum: Review of all possible options was not part of my purpose today, but revenue bonds were looked at and rejected based on debt capacity of the university. I could give you the whole study, but that's the short answer. Whether you or anyone else would have come to the same conclusions that we did is arguable. As a group we examined each of the options open to us, including revenue bonds and things of that nature.

If you have the debt capacity, which we did not have, it still raises the price of your product in a competitive market by an appreciable amount if you get a big bond issue.

Dr. Cecil Sheps: That's based on the assumption that the capital that comes from the for-profit chains does not require a return on its investment, which it clearly does – and generally more each year.

Mr. Philip Birnbaum: It can be spread across a larger base.

Quality

KURT DARR, SC.D, J.D., F.A.C.H.E.
Professor,
Department of Health Services Administration,
The George Washington University,
Washington, D.C.

Introductory Remarks: Status on the Quality of Care

As students in master's degree programs in hospital administration two decades ago, we were told unequivocally that by the early 1970s there would be no "proprietary hospitals." Their own greed and inappropriateness would have destroyed them. A few might remain in the southeast and southwest, but they would be small and of little significance; even if they somehow survived longer, it would make little difference. This was the heyday of the voluntary, not-for-profit, general acute care hospital. In the days before Medicare and Medicaid, it was queen of the health services system—a situation unlikely to ever recur.

The title of this section of the symposium is symptomatic of the problem that confronts both the for-profit and not-for-profit sectors of the health services system. At the extremes are those who argue that the profit motive is incompatible with delivery of high-quality care. They assert that there is an inherent conflict of interest between doing what is good for the patient and what is good for the bottom line and that delivery for health services is far too personal a thing to be achieved with an acceptable level of quality when consideration must be given to profit and shareholders. At the other extreme are those who assert that medical care is basically like any other service activity. They argue the customer must be served in the best way possible and that nothing is inherently contradictory in seeking to profit from such endeavors. They point to other service industries in which making profit is the norm. Indeed, a prominent example in our own field is that of the physician in a fee-for-service practice. In many ways, he is the archetypical businessman seeking to sell highly personalized services and earn a profit. Defenders of for-profit medicine argue that differences between the two are only superficial and that if the surface of the not-for-profit organization is scratched ever so lightly the apparent difference disappears. This argument is buttressed by the increasingly entrepreneurial spirit developing in the not-for-profit sector of the health services field.

This section addresses the quality of care delivered by for-profit and not-for-profit hospitals. This debate is substantially hindered by the paucity of data that compare quality of care in the two settings. The data available suggest there are no differences.

Although quality is easily defined as degree of adherence to preestablished criteria or standards, applying this in practice is quite difficult, if not impossible. Establishing standards requires thought and effort to determine what ends are sought and how they will be achieved. For the health services organization such as the hospital, this necessitates having not only criteria and standards, but systems and procedures that make it possible to compare actual against expected perfomance. These equally important elements of quality assurance activities require some means of surveillance to detect deviations and to ensure that corrective action is taken to improve performance. A crude analogy is the quality control activities performed in manufacturing and service industries. In many parts of health services settings, even the techniques are similar.

Donabedian has devoted a lifetime to questions surrounding quality of care issues in the health services field. His multi-volume series, *Exploration in Quality Assessment and Monitoring*, painstakingly identifies the problems of defining the quality of medical care and measuring the quality of the interpersonal relationship between physician and patient, which is essential to the process, and is reflected in the outcome of that care. The technical aspects of care are more definable and measurable. Regardless, any effort to measure quality begins with criteria, whether developed in-house, imposed from outside, or both.

Donabedian (1980) suggests that evaluation of quality of care can occur at three points in the delivery of medical services: structure, process, and outcome. He defines *structure* as the tools and resources that providers of care have at their disposal and the physical and organizational settings in which they work. *Process* is the set of activities that go on within and between practitioners and patients. Here judgment of quality may be made either by direct observation or by reviewing recorded information. Donabedian considers this means of measuring quality to be largely normative, in that the norms come either from the science of medicine or from the ethics and values of society. *Outcome* is a change in a patient's current and future health status that can be attributed to antecedent health care. This is defined very broadly and includes improvement of social and psychological function in addition to physiological aspects. Also included are patient attitudes, health-related knowledge acquired by the patient, and health-related behavioral change.

In comparing structure, process, and outcome, Donabedian concludes that "good structure, that is, a sufficiency of resources and proper system design, is probably the most important means of protecting and promoting the quality of care." (p. 82.) He adds, however, that assessment of structure is a good deal less important than assessment of process and outcome. Of the latter two, neither is clearly preferable. Each has advantages and disadvantages; most important, it is the link that can be established between the two that really counts–and, of course, the ability to replicate that link. Achieving a "good" outcome without knowing how it was done is knowing only part of the answer.

In the final analysis, results of efforts to measure (control) clinical and administrative quality must change behavior. Changing behavior is achieved through positive and negative means. Positive means include education, improvement of interpersonal relations and morale, as well as enhancing the structure to facilitate delivery of quality care. Negative means include sanctions against individuals and, in the case of programs such as prospective payment, financial risk to organizations. Generally, positive sanctions, especially education, are attempted first. There is evidence that in most cases in which the physician does not adhere to criteria, it is the result of conscious choice. In these situations, the physician knows what action is correct but does not take it. In such cases, education will be of no assistance for several reasons: the physician acted out of carelessness; the criteria were believed to lack legitimacy; the criteria were considered unimportant; the criteria were for some reason impossible to meet; or the physician acted intuitively or on the basis of experience and judgment. Similar problems likely exist with nonphysician professionals and management staff. Ultimately, it may be necessary for the hospital to take sanctions against the individual, even to the point their association is discontinued.

The two papers included in this section analyze the issues and problems involved in the comparison of the quality of care delivered in not-for-profit hospitals versus investor-owned hospitals. In "Quality of Care and For-Profit Hospitals," LoGerfo, who is affiliated with the not-for-profit sector, reviews previous studies of quality and for-profit ownership and concludes they are either outdated or that variance is inadequately explained by the data analyzed. He suggests that the issue is not whether profit will be generated, since both types of ownership must do so to survive; instead, the major issue is how. LoGerfo hypothesizes that organizations will assure themselves of profits either by shifting to product and service lines that are profitable or by various cost reduction strategies. In either case, there are significant policy implications of cost and quality trade-offs.

Studies comparing rates of caesarean sections performed by type of ownership show little difference between for-profit and not-for-profit private hospitals (Placek, P. J., Taffel, S., and Moien, M., 1983). There is a major difference, however, between private hospitals and publicly-owned hospitals. Of course, differences in rates alone do not support a conclusion that either type of hospital is acting appropriately. Indeed, both may be acting inappropriately. LoGerfo emphasizes the physician's importance in making resource allocation decisions for individual patients. He suggests the physician's independence will protect patients from dangerous cost reductions. In his opinion, it is more likely quality-sacrificing reductions will occur through restrictions on resources available to all patients, not to just a few.

LoGerfo's paper concludes with a brief discussion of strategies for maintaining quality. These emphasize the importance of research showing that greater physician involvement in management and governing body decisions is associated with higher quality of care. The visibility of decisions also is linked to higher quality of care. The paper ends by stressing the potentially positive effects on quality of vertical integration of health services delivery components; system-wide control activities that compare quality and managerial measures of performance; and designating a specific physician who supervises care in a given area of the hospital. Of course, these are potential attributes of all multi-hospital systems, regardless of ownership.

The second paper in this section, "How Does the Profit Motive Affect the Quality of Care?" is coauthored by Roeder and Moxley, who are both associated with a major for-profit multi-hospital system. Their paper focuses on the importance of medical staff in determining how resources are allocated and the quality of care achieved. A review of this literature and the research findings shows no striking differences between investor-owned and not-for-profit hospital, in terms of medical staff, organization, and involvement. The authors cite studies of the American Hospital Association (AHA) that found similar numbers of physician applications received, similar length of accreditation processes and probationary periods, and similar hospital requirements for board-certified physicians for both types of ownerships. They also cite studies by the American Medical Association showing few differences by ownership. Some distinctions found in one AHA study were that investor-owned hospitals have more physicians as voting members of hospital governing boards and executive committees, are less likely to have long range planning committees, are likely to have fewer medical staff committees in general, and are less likely to employ physicians or to bill directly for physician services.

The Roeder-Moxley paper identifies the presence of the new economic imperatives and decries the kind of broad brush approach taken in a reimbursement mechanism such as prospective payment. It discusses at length the importance of the market in identifying both price and value and the necessity for using this information in decision-making. Increasingly, consumers, acting on their own or represented by others who purchase health services for them, have learned to differentiate the value of a product or service. The authors strongly suggest that the consumer is also learning to make health services purchase decisions.

Beyond this increased awareness and sophistication lies the continuing problem of peer review. Studies of practice patterns consistently show significant variation in how physicians deliver medical care. Roeder and Moxley suggest that the new prospective payment system will exacerbate the problem previously encountered under cost reimbursement – that is, peer review bodies may not be asked to consider what more might have been done, but instead what less might be done. They conclude that reviewers will make complex and potentially life-threatening recommendations based only on their collective and habit-laden insights.

Roeder and Moxley note the presence of increasingly sophisticated and available patient care data bases that allow a better understanding of the relationship of particular practice patterns and outcomes in clinically similar cases. Development of systematic patient care information by both payers and providers will assist all parties in the treatment decision. They acknowledge, however, that, at worst, this could result in cookbook medicine – something initially suggested as a potential and highly undesirable result of the original professional standards review organization legislation in 1972. But at its best, it permits all parties to this critical transaction to be aware of input and output.

The most important aspect of the two papers in this section is that even though the authors are from divergent parts of the health services system, they reach the same conclusion: There are at present no data to support the position that investor-owned hospitals are inimical to the quality of care. Indeed, a large number of structure measures that compare the two groups show they are quite similar in most important respects. In addition, these papers isolate the issues especially germane to the future of health care quality regardless of ownership of the setting where it is delivered: the importance of adequate and properly applied data bases used by informed payers and consumers, and the necessity of effective medical staff-hospital interaction for cost and quality control.

REFERENCES

Donabedian, Avedis. *Explorations in Quality Assessment and Monitoring, Vol. I. The Definition of Quality and Approaches to its Assessment.* Ann Arbor, Michigan: Health Administration Press, 1980.

Placek, P. J., Taffel, S., and Moien, M. "Caesarean Section Delivery Rates: United States, 1981." *American Journal of Public Health,* 73(8): 861–862, August 1983.

JAMES P. LOGERFO, M.D., M.P.H.
Professor of Medicine and Health Services;
Co-Director, The Robert Wood Johnson
Clinical Scholars Program,
University of Washington
Schools of Medicine and
Public Health and Community Medicine

The Implications for Quality of Care

During the past decade, there has been a marked increase in the number and proportion of for-profit hospitals in the United States. The change has occurred primarily through new construction and purchase of existing facilities by investor-owned chains of hospitals. This has stimulated concern about the possible effect of for-profit ownership on the quality of patient care. Unfortunately, relatively few studies have been published on this particular topic. This paper attempts to present a framework for determining the effect of investor ownership on quality; to make some predictions about quality based on knowledge of other structural correlates of quality that tend to co-exist with for profit ownership of hospitals; and to identify possible strategies that might be used by any hospital trying to maintain or increase surplus revenue without lowering the quality of care.

To focus the discussion, it is important to review the relationships among the general population, disease, the medical care system, the care process, and health outcomes. These relationships are shown schematically in Figure 1. The ownership status of hospitals is considered to be a structural trait of the system. Thus, it will modulate health outcomes for patients by the extent to which it alters access to care and the extent to which it affects the care process for those patients who have gained entry. Structural traits affect the process of care both by setting maximum limits on the professional and technical resources available and by limiting or facilitating effective coordination of services.

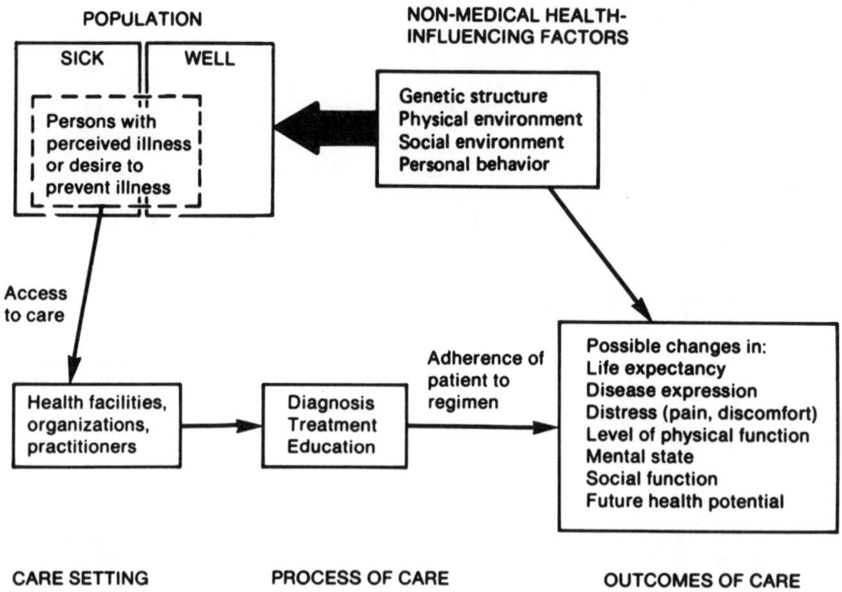

FIGURE 1. Model of a single episode of medical care.

PREVIOUS STUDIES OF QUALITY AND FOR-PROFIT OWNERSHIP

Since access to care is the subject of other papers in this symposium, I will focus instead on the quality of care for patients who have gained entry into the system. Because we are ultimately most concerned with health outcomes, I will first review data on the association between for-profit ownership and quality of care. Palmer and Reilly (1979) reviewed earlier studies of hospital characteristics and quality of care and could reach no firm conclusions about health outcomes and for-profit ownership. What few outcome data existed were from studies of hospitals in the 1960s or very early 1970s, and only a few studies adequately adjusted for case severity in the study hospitals. Forrest, Brown and Scott (1978) in the Institutional Differences Study (IDS) found a positive relationship between better standardized operative mortality ratios and proprietary or public, non-federal ownership compared to other hospitals. Interestingly, the same relationship was found for the ratio of registered nurses to licensed practical nurses, which has been higher in for-profit hospitals in recent years (Lewin, Derzon and Margulies, 1981). In contrast to the IDS study, Williams (1979) reported worse standardized perinatal mortality outcomes in for-profit hospitals than others, but only one percent of the variance was explained by for-profit ownership using data from 1965 to 1973. Given that so little variance was explained and that this was usually the last variable to enter the equations, it is not clear what significance should be attached to the findings. In addition, since the nature of the for-profit system is so radically different in 1984 than in 1975, no firm conclusion can be reached from existing literature about quality of care in the types of hospitals now dominating the for-profit sector compared to their non-profit counterparts.

PROFIT-MAXIMIZING STRATEGIES AND QUALITY

Given the lack of data about health outcomes, what issues should be considered for predicting the likely effects of the growing for-profit system on quality of care? Any formulation on how the structural element of "for-profit" might affect the health of patients actually seen will have to make predictions about the effect of "for-profit" ownership on the process of care. Before predicting such effects, however, it is important to consider how other structural aspects of care might also vary and interact with the structural element of "for-profit." When one looks at how other elements, such as payment systems or competition, affect an institution's ability to generate a profit, it becomes clear that how profit is generated will have a greater impact on quality than whether profit is generated and paid to investors. These concerns are generic to any institution that generates "profit," independent of whether the profits inure to investors or to the institution and its employees. The concerns may be magnified, however, when the need to generate profits for investors is added to the need to generate profit to support institutional improvements. Therefore, I will comment briefly on how profit can be generated and on how these alternatives might interact with quality of care. Those readers familiar with accounting theory will recognize that the following notions of profit and of how profit can be generated are quite simplistic, but they illustrate major concerns.

Hospitals can be viewed as businesses with a variety of product lines (e.g., cardiac surgery, obstetrical care) and a series of alternatives for managing a given illness (e.g., should a patient with a myocardial infarction be treated in the coronary care unit or in a routine ward?). At any given point, the "profit" (i.e., revenues minus cost) from the various product lines will vary. In a health system that has no constraints on the money available to pay for health care and in which there is no competition, profits can be readily generated by increasing prices. If total dollars become constrained or prices regulated, however, then profits can be ensured by shifting to those product lines that are profitable; by reducing the costs of producing any given service; and by targeting services to those purchasers that pay full cost, including cost for capital replacement and bad debt.

If the first strategy is chosen (i.e., shifting to profitable services only), then the concern for quality involves having an appropriate match between the medical needs and services available to the community. Such a strategy may hinder access directly by eliminating needed services or indirectly by competing successfully for patient groups necessary to the financial viability of other community hospitals that also provide some of the needed, but unprofitable, services. Nevertheless, a shift to services that are more profitable does not necessarily have negative implications for the quality of the services rendered. While subtle institutional pressures will exist to provide some of the services which are not clearly indicated (a negative effect), the consolidation may increase case volume for these services. The latter effect may be associated with better quality (Luft, Bunker and Enthoven, 1979).

The second strategy for increasing profits (i.e., lowering costs) can be achieved by reducing the per unit costs of existing labor, supplies, or fixed equipment; through increased productivity per unit; through subsitution of different, less costly units; or by a combination of these strategies. A summary of concerns regarding cost reduction strategies and quality of care is shown in Table 1. At present, based on existing data, it is as easy to argue for positive effects as for negative effects on quality for most of the cost reducing strategies. But since a possible cost-quality trade-off is a matter of great concern in considering ways to ensure profits, I will consider the matter in more detail, drawing on discussions from Donabedian et.al. (1982), and LoGerfo and Brook (1983).

QUALITY OF CARE AND COSTS OF CARE

In Figure 2, a cost-quality curve is shown for a given type of patient in a hospital. The Harmful curve represents care that either is inappropriate for patients – thereby exposing them to unnecessary risk – or that actually does more harm than good. In contrast, the Ideal curve shows that as costs go up, so do health benefits until

TABLE 1
Impact of Cost Containment on Quality of Care

Cost Reductions	Concerns Regarding Institutional Quality
Personnel	
Maintain same labor mix and productivity but negotiate lower salaries and benefits	Possible decrease in morale (loss of better workers)
Use different labor mix through substitution of lower paid workers for higher paid ones (e.g., Licensed Practical Nurses replacing Registered Nurses)	Loss of skill level may decrease quality (e.g., increased mistakes)
Increase productivity from current labor mix	Probably none but may affect morale.
Supplies/Drugs	
Negotiate lower prices for same supplies/drugs	None
Decrease supplies and drugs per patient	Possible underuse (undesirable) versus less overuse (desirable)
Change to less costly types of supplies and drugs	Possible decrease in effectiveness
Fixed Equipment	
Negotiate lower prices for same equipment	None
Increase unit productivity of current equipment to reduce need for purchase of more units (e.g., x-ray machines)	None (perhaps improved due to shorter length of stay)
Decrease use of need for fixed equipment (e.g., clinical protocols to decrease overuse)	Possible underuse versus less overuse (e.g., skull films in emergency room.

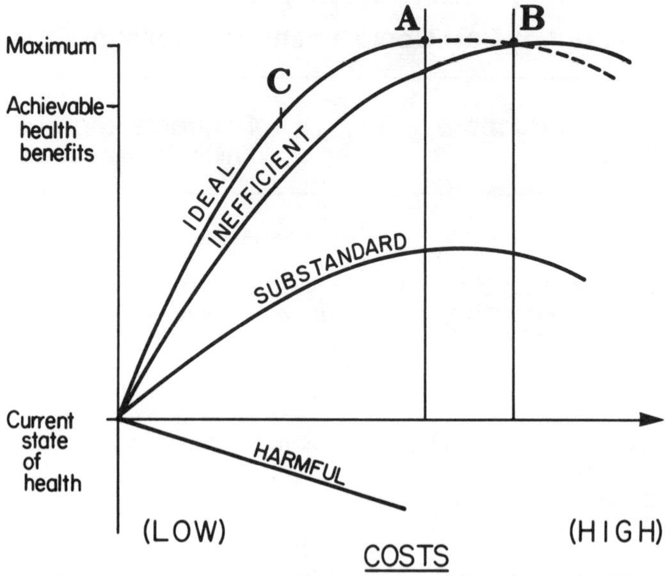

FIGURE 2. Relationship between quality as measured by health outcomes and costs of care.

point A. The ideal physician and hospital would stop at point A; however, some might provide quality-neutral services (shown by the dashed line), which increase costs to point B. Beyond point B, extra services become harmful (e.g., too many diagnostic tests lead to false-positive diagnoses). Note that some institutions might provide care on the Ideal curve, but due to resource limitation are never able to get to point A; this is represented by point C on the Ideal curve. The Inefficient curve represents a patient who achieves the same maximal benefit as the ideal setting but at a higher cost due to inefficiencies in production.

Those who argue that hospital costs can be reduced without sacrificing quality assume that hospitals are operating beyond point A on the Ideal curves or are operating on the Inefficient curve, since no one argues publicly for reducing quality. The claims that for-profit hospitals are more efficient than other hospitals are also based on this assumption.

Unfortunately, we do not have adequate case-severity-adjusted data to state whether for-profit hospitals are closer to point A than point B on the Ideal curve or whether they are operating nearer the Ideal curve than the Inefficient curve when compared to non-profit hospitals. While the studies of costs per case in for-profit suggest a higher cost, we do not have adequate measures of case-severity to say with certainty that the costs were not related to case mix (Lewin, Derzon and Margulies, 1981; Pattison and Katz, 1983). For instance, Pattison and Katz attempted to adjust for case-mix severity through use of peer group assignment in California. While the peer-group assignment might encompass a measure of intensity of services commonly used, it may not adequately adjust for clinical severity of the cases nor for other factors causing different levels of clinically necessary services. Despite the inadequacy of case-severity adjustments, however, it is noteworthy that both major published studies about cost/case show a trend consistent with the notion that for-profits are somewhere to the right of other hospitals on cost axis, but it is not known where they lie with respect to quality of care. In this regard, the studies of Flood et.al. (1979) suggested better outcomes with higher intensity of services using only crude case-severity adjustments. Therefore, to the extent that higher charges per case in for-profit hospitals are related to more services per case, rather than just higher prices, it is possible that the quality of care is better.

Observations suggesting that for-profit hospitals may favor clinical strategies not based on need of patients can be found in Placek et. al.'s study (1983) of the rates of caesarean sections (C-sections). Data from their report are adapted in Table 2. Note that in the United States and each of the four regions, the rates of caesarean sections are higher in the for-profit hospitals than in the public hospitals. In all but the South, the rates of this operation are higher in for-profit than in voluntary hospitals. Also, the rates are higher in aggregate and in virtually all of the source-of-pay versus region interactions. These data suggest (but do not prove) that the "for-profit" trait is an independent marker for unnecessarily high rates of caesarean sections. If one believes that for-profit hospitals get a more complex obstetrical mix – such as a significantly higher portion of women over age 35 or women with prior caesarean sections – then the higher rates might be appropriate. This possibility has been partially explored by Williams and Chen (1983) who found no difference between voluntary, private hospitals and for-profit hospitals, but they explored only primary C-section rates. While there was no difference among private, non-profit, and for-profit hospitals, the public hospitals had a much lower adjusted rate. This finding underscores my belief that although a public private dichotomy exists, there may be little difference between hospital behavior and type of ownership in the private sector.

TABLE 2
Caesarean Sections per 100 Births, 1981

	Nation-wide	West	South	North	Central
Northeast Ownership					
Proprietary	22	22.5	18.9	30.4	25.5
Public	15.4	15.5	15.8	14.5	14.9
Voluntary	18.8	17.4	20.4	15.9	20.4
Payer Source					
Self-pay	14.4	15.1	15.0	11.3	14.9
Medicaid	16.1	17.7	15.9	15.3	16.1
Blue Cross	20.2	17.9	23.3	17.4	21.1
Commercial	18.7	17.7	19.6	16.8	22.7

From: Placek, P. J., Taffel, S., and Moien, M. "Caesarean Section Delivery Rates: United States, 1981" *American Journal of Public Health*, 73(8): 861–862, August, 1983.

Even though there is concern that a desire for increased profits will prompt some providers to reduce both cost and quality, there is no published evidence to indicate that for-profit hospitals will respond in this manner rather than shifting to more profitable types of care to ensure a profit. Given the relative independence of physicians from direct administrative control and their fiduciary obligation to patients, it is unlikely that such dangerous cost reduction will be readily identifiable in decisions about the care of individual patients. More likely, quality-sacrificing reductions would occur on a wider basis through restrictions of resources available to all patients (e.g., cutbacks in nursing or restricted hours for use of computerized axial tomography scanning). This is reflected in point C on Figure 2.

If physicians are totally autonomous within the resource limitations of a given hospital, then questions arise as to whether they will change to cost-reducing – or revenue-enhancing – behaviors that are in the hospital's best interest. Despite their semi-independence, it is clear that physicians will alter behavior to some extent in a manner favorable to the hospital. This was evident in the way in which length-of-stay changes occurred in New York compared to Pennsylvania when different prospective payment projects were implemented in the early 1970s. The mean length-of-stay changed in directions favorable to the hospitals in each state, but in different directions in each state. Thus, it may be naive to believe that physicians' fiduciary relationships to patients will not be modified somewhat to serve the interests of the hospitals. This tendency will become greater as increased competition forces hospitals and physicians to establish closer, joint risk-taking arrangements.

STRATEGIES TO MAINTAIN QUALITY

Given the importance of the medical staff-hospital interaction in controlling costs and quality, under what circumstances might medical staffs be more responsive to institutional concern about cost restrictions and how might these relate to quality? In general, one would predict that tightly organized medical staffs comprising key people with strong institutional commitment (e.g., partially salaried or other contractual arrangement) would be most responsive to a hospital's interests. Interestingly, these same characteristics may also be associated with a higher level of care. For instance, hospitals with medical staff representation on governing boards and decision-making groups have been found to provide better care (Shortell and LoGerfo, 1981). In this regard, it is noteworthy that for-profit chains of hospitals have been found to have a higher percentage of physicians and inside managers on corporate-level boards than non-profit hospital chains (Derzon, Lewin and Watt, 1981). Also, hospitals with higher internal visibility of consequences have been associated with better hospital performance. Consistent with this notion is the observation by Williams of a positive relationship between the presence of a perinatal morbidity review committee and lower standardized perinatal mortality rates (Williams, 1979). Certainly, increased visibility of consequences of decision making will by a *sine qua non* of a hospital that is trying to maintain a high level of quality yet increase staff sensitivity to cost issues within the hospital.

With respect to visibility of consequences, for-profit hospitals that are part of chains have the potential advantage of being able to develop quality control systems that allow for comparison among their own hospitals on case-severity-adjusted quality measures, as well as on financial measures. If used appropriately, hospitals with lower quality will be readily identifiable, and presumably, remedial actions will occur. An added incentive for chain members to protect quality of care is that one or two bad hospitals in a system have the potential to tarnish the reputation of the entire chain. Of course, this is true of any chain system, including non-profit chains.

Based on data from existing literature, I believe those hospitals that can most effectively institute concurrent feedback systems using contingency-based care strategies will be the most successful at maintaining quality while reducing costs. If hospitals try to cut costs by discretionary rationing of care on a case-by-case basis, without sacrificing quality, they will need key clinicians with strong commitment to oversee the process. For instance, if one were to try to optimize the use of intensive care unit of a hospital with a large, diverse staff, it would likely require the presence of one or two physicians who could help allocate the beds to patients clearly in need and encourage transfer as soon as it is safe for those already in the unit. The physician presence would be necessary for the process to be acceptable to the medical staff. Thus, one would expect greater medical staff participation in setting institutional policy. The same type of argument will probably apply to other cost-cutting measures, such as decisions on how to restrict a drug formulary to decrease drug costs without sacrificing quality. In my experience, the decision to designate a physician to supervise care in a given area of the hospital where there has been relative autonomy of physicians is met initially with great reluctance, but long-term accomodation usually is achieved.

While the preceding discussion has emphasized cost-quality issues for hospitalized patients, it is important to note that one could lower hospital costs without decreasing quality by the development of vertically integrated systems of care – e.g., hospital care, ambulatory care, long-term care and home health care. Under a reimbursement system analogous to the diagnosis-related groups system, a hospital could arrange to decrease costs per case, yet maintain revenues and quality by earlier discharge to lower levels of care within the same system. If those lower levels of care also have the potential to generate profits for the system to which the hospital belongs, then profit will be maintained despite loss of total revenue. This could permit both plant equipment renewal and payment of investors. For example, a home-care intravenous program could be instituted for osteomyelitis patients and supervised home dialysis could be used more extensively for patients with kidney disease.

The potential to develop such vertical systems – either by ownership or contractual agreement – is not restricted to for-profit institutions, but their greater access to capital may give the for-profits greater mobility in this direction. The tendency to move toward vertical systems will be greatly enhanced by any system of reimbursement using capitation payments, again reflecting the critical role of other aspects of the financial and competitive structure of the health system in predicting likely effects of for-profit systems on quality of care.

Indeed, no clear conclusions can be drawn about quality of care for patients who have access to hospital care and the increased role of for-profit hosptials in the United States. However, since concerns have been raised about access to care, and since access will modulate quality at the societal level, some comments are in order about selected aspects of the access issue.

As in previous discussions, the reader will note that one would predict no major trend difference between access to for-profit versus private, voluntary institutions in a competitive environment, but perhaps an exaggerated trend would occur in the former to restrict access for non-profitable patient groups. In any event, to the extent that for-profits restrict access to care, they are likely to do so for those populations with low incomes covered by public programs when full costs are not paid and for uninsured low-income patients. To the extent that profit-maximizing services are provided and that other services needed by the community are not provided by the for-profits, then other institutions will have to provide those ignored services if quality is to remain intact. This could result in some duplication of services and facilities that may ultimately increase total societal costs of care, independent of how it is financed, since the non-profit hospitals will duplicate some profitable services to be viable. The resulting cost increase to society may subsequently reduce the willingness to support public programs or hospitals. If so, then access is likely to be further reduced for those who require public support, but the reduction will occur indirectly, and not just in care given by the for-profit institutions. Such reductions will decrease quality at the societal level.

Clearly, the net impact of for-profits will be inextricably intertwined with public decisions concerning whether the level of care construed as a societal responsibility by the President's Commission on Ethics in Biomedical Research (1983) will be accepted or rejected. If rejected, quality of care, for the nation as a whole, will suffer.

REFERENCES

Cummins, R. O., LoGerfo, Inui, T. S., et. al. "High Yield Referral Criteria for Post-Traumatic Skull Roentgenography." *Journal of the American Medical Association*, 244 (7):673–676, August 15, 1980.

Derzon, R. A., Lewin, L. S., and Watt, J. M. "Not-for-profit Chains Share in Multihospital System Boom." *Hospitals*, 55(10):65–71, May 16, 1981.

Donabedian, A., Wheeler, J. R. C., and Wyszewianski, L. "Quality, Cost and Health." *Medical Care*, 20(10):975–992, October 1982.

Flood, A. B., Ewy, W., Scott, W. R., Forrest, W. H., and Brown, B. W. "The Relationship Between Intensity and Duration of Medical Services and Outcomes for Hospitalized Patients." *Medical Care*, 17(11):1088–1102, November 1979.

Forrest, W. H., Brown, B. W., Scott, W. R., Ewy, W., and A. B. Flood. "Impact of Hospital Characteristics on Surgical Outcomes and Length of Stay: Final Report to National Center for Health Services Research." Washington, D.C.: U.S. Government Printing Office, 1978. (DHHS, HRA, 230–75–0173).

Lewin, L. S., Derzon, R. A., and Margulies, R. "Investor-Owneds and Non-profits Differ in Economic Performance." *Hospitals*, 55(13):52–58, July 1, 1981.

LoGerfo, J. P. and Brook, R. "Assessing and Assuring the Quality of Medical Care." In William, S. (ed.) *Health Services and Medical Care, Volume II*. New York: John Wiley, 1983.

Luft, H., Bunker, J. P. and Enthoven, A. C. "Should Operations be Regionalized?" *The New England Journal of Medicine*, 301(25):1364–1369, December 20, 1979.

Palmer, R. H., Reilly, M. and Reilly, C. "Individual and Institutional Variables Which May Serve as Indicators of Quality of Medical Care." *Medical Care*, 17(7):693–717, July 1979.

Pattison, R. V. and Katz, H. M. "Investor-Owned and Not-for-profit Hospitals: A Comparison Based on California Data." *The New England Journal of Medicine*, 309(10):347–353, August 11, 1983.

Placek, P. J., Taffel, S., and Moien, M. "Caesarean Section Delivery Rates: United States, 1981." *American Journal of Public Health*, 73(8):861–862, August 1983.

President's Commission for the Study of Ethical Problems in Medicine and Biomedical and Behavioral Research. "Securing

Access to Health Care: Volume One Report." Washington, D.C.: Government Printing Office, 1983.

Rehm, S. J. and Weinstein, A. J. "Home Intravenous Antibiotic Therapy: a Team Approach." *Annals of Internal Medicine*, 99(3):388–392, September 1983.

Shortell, S. M. and LoGerfo, J. P. "Hospital Medical Staff Organization and Quality of Care: Results for Myocardial Infarction and Appendectomy." *Medical Care*, 19(10):1041–1053, October 1981.

Williams, R. L. "Measuring the Effectiveness of Perinatal Medical Care." *Medical Care*, 17(2):95–109, February 1979.

William, R. L. and Chen, P. M. "Controlling the Rise in Caesarean Section Rates by Dissemination of Information from Vital Records." *American Journal of Public Health*, 73(8):863–867, August 1983.

PENELOPE C. ROEDER
Assistant Vice President,
American Medical International, Inc.

JOHN H. MOXLEY III, M.D.
Senior Vice President,
American Medical International, Inc.

How Does the Profit Motive Affect the Quality of Care?

Quality of care is not a new concern for the American health care system, but it has never been as pervasive a concern as it now is under prospective pricing. Until recently, it was generally assumed that quality care was available in direct proportion to the resources available. As a result, quality issues generally have been raised only in regard to groups recognized to have limited resources available for health care – the elderly and the poor.

Under cost reimbursement, there has been little, if any, relationship between the institutional profit motive and the quality of care delivered to most patients. The American health care system has heretofore afforded almost unobstructed expression to the professional model by supporting nearly absolute professional discretion (Light, 1983). With relatively few constraints on available financial resources, health care professionals – generally physicians – have been free to prescribe whatever care they thought advisable with little concern about reimbursement.

In that environment, most studies of quality have focused primarily on the *process* of delivering care. Despite Dr. E. A. Cod-

(Some of the material in this paper is adopted from, "Promoting Quality Care in Cost-Effective Settings." *Business and Health*, 2 (3): 30–31, January/February 1985.)

man's plea in 1913 that quality of care should be measured by examining health care admissions one year after treatment (Codman, 1914), many analysts have instead focused on a variety of input and structural measures in their studies of quality care. Since most studies have focused on hospital care, many of the proxies rely on institutional factors such as staffing patterns and governance (Palmer and Reilly, 1979). The studies often rely heavily on the retrospective examination of patient records. Consequently, these studies frequently use in-hospital mortality rates or other short-term mortality and morbidity rates as the measure of quality (Shortell and LoGerfo, 1981). In addition, these retrospective studies have many of the problems attendant on research that lacks an *a priori* protocol (Moss, 1981).

Because of the growing interest in the for-profit hospital industry, there have been a number of recent studies comparing quality of care in investor-owned hospitals with the care in not-for-profit facilities. Although these studies rely on the traditional methodologies and proxy measures, they reveal some interesting findings.

The first such study compares medical staff size and hospital privileges and compensation arrangements. It was drawn from the 1982 American Hospital Association (AHA) Survey of Medical Staff Organization and the 1982 AHA Validation Survey of Multi-Hospital Systems. The study controlled for system size, hospital size, teaching activity, geographic region, and size of each facility's Standard Metropolitan Statistical Area. It indicated the following: there is no difference in the number of physician applications received by investor-owned versus not-for-profit hospitals, although investor-owned hospitals accept a larger percentage of applications; there is no difference in the length of either the accreditation processes or the probationary periods in the privileging processes at investor-owned and not-for-profit hospitals; and there are no differences in the various types of hospital requirements regarding board certification or the number of board-certified physicians per 100 beds (Morrisey, Alexander and Shortell, 1984).

Another study based on AHA data focused on physician participation in the administrations and governments of hospitals. In general, the study showed that the characteristics of medical staffs of investor-owned and not-for-profit hospitals are not strikingly different. Interestingly, investor-owned hospitals have more physicians as voting members of the hospital governing boards and their executive committees; investor-owned hospitals are less likely to have long-range planning committees and more likely to have fewer medical staff committees in general; and investor-owned hospitals are less likely to employ physicians or to direct-bill for physician services (Alexander, Morrisey and Shortell, 1984).

Data from the American Medical Association's (AMA) 1984 Socioeconomic Monitoring Systems Core Survey and its 1984 Physician Opinion Survey tended to confirm these findings. In addition, the AMA data indicated that there were only slight differences in the number of years since hospital medical staffs had completed their residencies, in the amount of time per patient physicians spent in the hospital, and in perceptions of nursing support and patient satisfaction. The most significant difference found in the AMA surveys was not between investor-owned and not-for-profit hospital staffs, but between public hospitals and all private sector facilities (SMS Report, 1984).

Although the appropriateness of these proxies for the quality of care may be questioned, most of the evidence tends to support the conclusion that the tax status of provider institutions has little effect on the quality of care in the cost-based reimbursement environment.

The cost-reimbursement era has now ended. Medicare has introduced the diagnosis-related group (DRG) based prospective pricing system; the number of enrollees in capitated payment health care systems is rising; and American industry has announced its intention to become "prudent purchasers" of health care. In short, the American health care system is now confronted by a general limitation on resources. Recognition that the role of economic imperatives may be significantly different in this new environment has fueled growing concern about the quality of care.

The introduction of the new, more stringent economic imperatives is often attributed to the presence and growth of the investor-owned health care companies. However, as Eli Ginzberg (1984) points out, the development of health care as a business is itself an outgrowth of the "monetarization" of health care that began before the widespread adoption of hospital insurance in the 1950s. That expansion of hospital insurance; the growth of government financing for the capital expansion of health care facilities, medical education, and research; and the programs created by the Social Security amendments of 1965 have all contributed to the growing importance of the economic incentives in the American health care system.

The pros and cons of introducing economic incentives into the health delivery system have been widely debated. Interestingly, that debate often focuses only on hospital care. Medicare's DRG system, along with many other prospective pricing systems, is directed toward cutting the cost of hospitalization. Unless that focus is broadened, the best that can be anticipated under prospective pricing is more efficient hospital care. While more efficient hospitalization may be desirable, it has no known relationship to health care outcomes.

From a quality-of-care perspective, this type of simplistic approach to health care cost reduction may indeed be detrimental to the American health care consumer. Any system that focuses on reducing the cost of each incident of care may contain incentives that ignore the possibility of long-term costs. Thus, such systems may reward ineffective but repeated treatment or ineffective treatment that creates a greater demand for more intensive chronic care.

It is hoped, however, that the new "prudent purchasers" of health care – be they the Federal Government or private sector industrial concerns – will recognize that they must broaden their focus beyond individual incidents of care to total case management. Only if they begin to view health care delivery as an ongoing process, requiring a variety of settings over a period of time, can they succeed in reducing their long-term costs.

Private sector health care purchasers are well aware that the American economy is not a simple price-driven economy. Unlike a pure commodities market, the marketplace is filled with differentiable products. As a result, the economy is increasingly value-driven. A small sampling of recent television advertising indicates that the sellers of most small durables believe that consumers are at least as concerned about perceived value as they are about price.

A quarter century of research into the quality of medical care provided by different groups or in different settings suggests that health care is also a differentiable product. The same companies that have learned to sell value can be expected to learn to buy it. The economic interests of those large purchasers of health care will force providers to learn what the rest of American industry has already learned – that product is very important in a competitive environment.

With the advent of market incentives in health care, these large purchasers can create a market in which quality of care is the only thing that allows a provider to stay in business. The information systems needed to collect and analyze data relating to quality of care are as readily available to large purchasers of health care as they are to providers. When making claims of quality or cost-effectiveness, providers will increasingly be called on to provide specific evidence to expert buyers and analysts.

These are not only academic or hypothetical issues; they are real, important, and complex operating issues. Take, for example, the case of Stanford University Medical Center. Most would agree that all the inpatient services at Stanford provide high-quality care. A recent study revealed that costs for high-risk patients on the faculty services were nearly 70 percent higher than for similar patients on the community services, after adjusting for case mix. The in-hospital mortality rate for the higher cost faculty services was lower than the in-hospital mortality rate for the less expensive community services. However, nine months after discharge, the mortality rates for the patients on the faculty services and the community service were virtually identical (Garber, Fuchs and Silverman, 1984). In economic terms, the additional cost bought an incremental nine months of life.

How does one judge whether that nine months was worth the 70% cost differential? Certainly, that judgment must take into account the patients, the quality of their lives during the nine months, and the non-dollar cost associated with the "extra" diagnostic procedures and treatments (e.g., pain, disfigurement). Even leaving aside all those very important questions, it is impossible to avoid the fact that the physicians, the patients, and the payers involved probably did not have the medical information necessary to help decide which course was right for them at the time – in other words, what their trade-offs were.

Traditionally, treatment decisions have been the sole province of physicians. However, recent studies have shown that practice patterns are subject to considerable variation (Wennberg, 1982). Some analysts impute the differences to "style," (Wennberg, 1984) while others argue that habit and conservatism are significant (Linzer, 1984; Doubilet and Abrams, 1984). All these factors probably play roles, as do the institutional factors that reinforce them – the various peer review organizations that have dominated the professional model American health care system.

Cost-reimbursement, peer review organizations, including hospital review committees and Professional Standards Review Organizations, considered such questions as what might have been done wrong, what more might have been done to save a patient, and how a particular case was different from so-called normal cases. In answering these questions, the peer reviewers had nothing more objective than their collective experience and their own definitions of "normal" and "necessary" on which to rely. Furthermore, they had to provide definitions of "normal" and "necessary." Moreover, by focusing on aberrant cases, the review processes contributed little to the understanding of these terms.

Prospective pricing has added a new dimension to these activities: peer review bodies may no longer be asked to consider what more might have been done for a patient, but instead what less might have been done. The reviewers will be called on to make complex and potentially life-threatening recommendations based only on their collective and habit-laden insights. They have little if any objective, data-based information about the clinical links between the indications for use and the outcomes for most common procedures (Brook et. al., 1984).

It is the infusion of economic incentives into the health care systems that makes the creation of the massive data systems needed for this kind of research plausible. The development of high-speed, low-cost computers made possible the manipulation of large data sets. However, the relative independence of each of the many providers and payers that form the health care system mitigated against systematic collection of the necessary data. In the current more stringent economic environment, both payers and providers have strong incentives to manage costs and both groups need data to achieve that objective.

To manage patients in a clinically appropriate manner, providers need a body of clinical data. They cannot rely on DRG data because the discharge diagnosis does not help them understand how a physician should guide a patient from presentation through diagnosis to treatment. Many institutional providers (including St. Vincent's Hospital in Worcester, Massachusetts; Lutheran Hospital and Homes Society in Wells Fargo, North Dakota; and American Medical International) have, therefore, turned to systems based on clinical data obtained when a patient presents for treatment (Brown and Kloss, 1984). This kind of system allows providers to use standard clinical data to assign patients to groups according to type and severity of presenting complaint. Care can then be monitored by severity group.

In the earliest stages, these monitoring systems will support no conclusions. However they will allow identification of norms for each group using much of the same patient information data that now drives medical records reimbursement systems and DRG monitoring systems. Analysts will be able to identify average lengths-of-stay for each severity group. Within each of the groups, they can also identify average costs and ancillary utilization, as well as variations in those patterns.

With that information, analysts can begin to answer some of the questions of researchers: Are variations in physicians' response to a particular type of case due to some clinical factor to which attention is not often paid? Or do these variations result from a particular physician's or group of physicians' habit or style of practice? Over a period of time, the data also will yield a better understanding of the relation of particular practice patterns to outcomes in clinically similar cases.

The development of systematic patient care information by both payers and providers will assist all the parties who are now involved in treatment decisions. It will enable them to see what their options are and how they relate to both practice norms and outcome probabilities. At its worst, this could result in cookbook medicine (Burnham, 1984). However, used well, patient care information could be a very important tool. No two patients and no two cases will ever be identical; deviations from the norm will always occur. Well-constructed data bases will enable physicians to know what the norm is and how to get from point A to point B in the simplest manner in the majority of cases. Where the simplest solution is judged not to be the best solution the physician, the patient and the payer will know the relative risks, benefits, and costs of the alternatives. All parties can then make rational, logical choices (Wennberg and Gittelsohn, 1982).

These systems are not intended to be used by financial administrators to set arbitrary standards for health care practices. They are designed to be administered by health care professionals and intended to assist them in understanding first *how* health care is delivered and, ultimately, *why*. By encouraging that understanding, perhaps providers will modify their habits so that they provide quality care without unnecessary or redundant care. Modifying practice patterns will not be a simple or a rapid process. However, there is already evidence that physicians do respond to information about practice patterns by changing their style (Caper and Zubcoff, 1984).

The findings from the new data also may raise important and unexpected questions about efficient and effective health care. Many of those questions may demand carefully structured formal research. Solutions may require major changes in medical school curricula, health facility planning, and health insurance design. These are health system issues that can neither be ignored nor dealt with in isolation. It is hoped that the payers whose more stringent economic demands on providers are now forcing changes in practice patterns will recognize the value of obtaining all the information necessary to support long-term cost-effective changes in the health care system.

The American health care system has entered a new era. There is no question that the introduction of economic incentives will lead to some efficiencies. It continues, however, to be an open question whether those efficiencies will enhance or erode the quality of care.

The demands of cost management create an opportunity to develop lower cost delivery mechanisms. If payers and patients choose to demand long-term value rather than short-term efficiencies, the provider community will respond by learning how to measure and provide cost-effective, quality care.

REFERENCES

Alexander, Jeffrey A., Morrisey, Michael A., and Shortell, Stephen M. "Physician Participation in the Administration and Governance of System and Freestanding Hospitals: A Comparison by Type of Ownership." Working paper, Hospital Research and Educational Trust, AHA, September 1984.

Brook, Robert H. et. al. "Geographic Variations in the Use of Services: Do They Have Any Clinical Significance?" *Health Affairs,* 3(2):63–71, Summer 1984.

Brown, David L. and Kloss, Linda L. "Systemwide QA Leans Heavily on Board Talk! Lutheran Hospital and Homes Society's QA Network is Structured Around Interfacility Communications." *Multis*, 2(2):42–50, Summer 1984.

Burnham, John F. "The Unfortunate Case of Dr. Z: How to Succeed in Medical Practice in 1984." *The New England Journal of Medicine*, 310(11):729–30, March 15, 1984.

Caper, Philip and Zubcoff, Michael. "Managing Medical Cost Through Small Area Analysis." *Business and Health*, 1(9):20–25, September 1984.

Codman, E. A. "The Product of a Hospital." *Surgery, Gynecology and Obstetrics*, 18(4):491–496, April, 1914.

Doubilet, Peter and Abrams, Herbert L. "The Cost of Underutilization: Percutaneous Transterminal Angioplasty for Peripheral Vascular Disease." *The New England Journal of Medicine*, 310(2):95–102, January 12, 1984.

Garber, Alan M., Fuchs, Victor R., and Silverman, James F. "Case Mix, Costs, and Outcomes: Differences Between Faculty and Community Services in a University Hospital." *The New England Journal of Medicine*, 310(19):1231–1237, May 10, 1984.

Ginzberg, Eli. "The Monetarization of Medical Care." *The New England Journal of Medicine*, 310(19):1162–1165, May 10, 1984.

Light, Donald W. "Is Competition Bad?" *The New England Journal of Medicine*, 309(21):1315–1318, November 24, 1983.

Linzer, Mark. "Doing What 'Needs' to be Done." *The New England Journal of Medicine*, 310(7):469–470, February 16, 1984.

Morrisey, Michael A., Alexander, Jeffrey A., Shortell, Stephen M. "Medical Staff Size, Hospital Privileges and Compensation Arrangements: A Comparison of System Hospitals." Working paper, Hospital Research and Educational Trust, AHA, September 1984.

Moss, Lincoln E. "The Series of Consecutive Cases as a Device for Assessing Outcomes of Intervention." *The New England Journal of Medicine*, 311(11):705–710, September 13, 1984.

Palmer, R. H. and Reilly, M. C. "Individual and Institutional Variables Which May Serve as Indicators of Quality of Medical Care." *Medical Care*, 17(7):693–717, July 1979.

"Profit in Medicine: The Impact on Hospital Staffing Patterns and Physician Practice Behavior." SMS Report, AMA Center for Health Policy Research, 3(4), June 1984.

Shortell, Stephen M. and LoGerfo, James P. "Hospital Medical Staff Organization and Quality of Care: Results for Myocardial Infarction and Appendectomy." *Medical Care*, 19(10):1041–1053, October 1981.

Wennberg, John E. "Should the Cost of Insurance Reflect the Cost of Use in Local Hospital Markets?" *The New England Journal of Medicine*, 307(22):1374–1381, November 25, 1982.

Wennberg, John E. "Dealing with Medical Practice Variations: A Proposal for Action." *Health Affairs*, 3(2):6–32, Summer 1984.

Wennberg, John and Gittelsohn, Alan. "Variations In Medical Care Among Small Areas." *Scientific American*, 246(4):120–134, April 1982.

Discussion – Quality

Dr. Bradford Gray, *Senior Professional Associate, Institute of Medicine*: I have been interested in the implications of the growth of the for-profit sector for research, and the tool that Dr. Moxley described intrigues me. I can imagine it being used in a number of ways. For example, would it be used to do studies within AMI hospitals that would be published in the literature? Would the methodology be published, or would the methodology that you are talking about essentially be proprietary? Can you imagine the company developing outcome statistics that would be used, for example, for advertising purposes? A lot of questions arise about how that might be used. I do not mean to imply anything by my question, but this topic intrigues me.

Dr. John H. Moxley III, *Senior Vice President, American Medical International, Inc.*: I do not take any implication other than curiosity.

I think that the reason we are doing it is because clearly things are changing around us just as they are for everybody else. We realize that the new circumstances are going to be different. What we are finding is that there is an interest in moving forward. I would think that this would not be proprietary information. I would think that quality data would be information that would be collected in a systematic way that would be available for investigators to look at, obviously, in the appropriate screened fashion so that specific identities would not be revealed.

Brad, I would hope that we would never come to a point where it would be used for advertising, because that certainly is not what it is intended for. I see quality measurements being used, quite frankly, to attempt to adjust to a new system in the most positive way, to provide care sufficiently without eroding quality. I think those are the desires.

Dr. Gary Filerman, *President, AUPHA*: One of the very significant factors in quality of care, as Jim mentioned, is the relationship between the physician and the factors that control the environment of practice.

Now, perhaps it is not a characteristic of only the for-profit sector, but one could certainly look at large scale multi-institutional organizations as holding out the possibility that administrative distance will become greater. That is, the individual physician will increasingly encounter constraints which do not originate at the level of the institution but are systematic and originate in Knoxville or in Detroit. Could you not see that leading to physicians organizing in a union-like fashion to protect what they consider to be the necessary conditions for medical care quality?

Dr. John H. Moxley III: The union in California, which I have observed for the last ten years, is currently sending letters to every physician in the country expanding things beyond that which you are talking about. They are saying, look, there is just no question, bad things are going to happen, they are going to be driven by HCFA (Health Care Financing Administration) and you are not going to be able to deal with them unless you are unionized. Please send in your initiation dues to so and so in Los Angeles, California.

Those of us in the California Medical Association have been getting those for ten years, now everybody in the AMA or everybody that they can get the name of is getting such letters. So I think that there is a mental set among a group of physicians who take the position that the only way they are going to survive as independent practitioners of medicine in the future is to formally form themselves into a union.

Dr. James LoGerfo, *Professor of Medicine and Health Services, University of Washington*: The systemic issue is there for the nonprofit, as well. For instance, one of my clinical scholars a few years ago was interested in racial differences and intensity of services around the country, so we used the Flood and Scott data sets. What was interesting to us was that it is clear, if one looks just at the severity of illness for some common things like pneumonia, that the intensity of services provided to blacks in the U.S. was lower than the intensity of services to other patients from their 2,400 hospital sample.

That was purely a function of the hospitals they were admitted to. If you look within each institution, the intensity of service was very similar. The problem was they had access, in general, to very different institutions, when looked at nationally. They were going to hospitals which gave lower intensity of services. You saw a reflection of that in the controversy at Harlem Hospital about getting a CT scanner. So, there are systemic problems within the public and nonprofit system, already, and this would be just a further reflection of that.

Dr. John H. Moxley III: I understand the full thrust of your question, but again, data that was reviewed briefly and that I had, but did not review, because of its redundancy, showed that the systematic control, if anything, seems to be less in investor-owned. The physicians in the investor-owned hospital seem to have a more arm's length relationship with whatever is going on than those that are not in investor-owned hospitals.

Dr. Gary Filerman: Well, the point that Dick Egdahl and others have made is that there are good times and there are bad times. One could look ahead to tougher times when organizational values might very well clash with the ideal conditions of the individual practitioner, who then would respond in different kinds of ways, such as responding collectively.

Dr. Bryan Luce, *Human Affairs Research Center, Battelle Memorial Institute*: I want to address the issue of quality in terms of some of the values that Dean Mott brought out in the beginning.

I think it is important that we think of where we are coming from and the way the values have been in the old system. There has been a lot of talk of physicians and evidence of physicians protecting their income. The AMA really has become self-serving in a lot of its actions. Anyone who has been in hospitals knows the old system of values where there was reluctance to give information to patients.

There have been problems with the old system. When you think in terms of new incentives and business orientation to health, you have to consider informing the consumer, making sure the consumer understands what his choices are, assuring him that there are choices, and hoping at least that the competitive environment and the new business orientation can be used to foster a more responsive system.

Dr. Basil J. F. Mott, *Dean, School of Health Studies, University of New Hampshire*: I think one of the interesting things, at least from my perspective, is how these two sets of values will work together in the long run. As you pointed out, there probably are some real benefits in terms of improving physician relations with patients and other things as a result of changes in the marketplace. But the other part of the question that interests me and maybe Dr. Moxley is to what extent are we in a situation where the behavior of each side is strongly influenced by the other?

We talk a good deal about the extent to which the nonprofits and voluntary hospitals are influenced by our new environment. To what extent do investor-owned hospitals feel influenced by the fact that they are in an environment that has essentially been voluntary and has a reservoir of basic values, and to what extent is that good or bad from their perspective?

Dr. John H. Moxley III: Well, I certainly think we feel all of those pressures as a group of organizations that are responsible for something like ten percent of the hospital beds in the country. Investor ownership of health facilities certainly has been receiving more attention over the last year, and it continues on.

I think what we are seeing, and I think this is being brought out in the data that are being reviewed is that, in fact, the pressures upon private hospitals, be they voluntary or investor-owned, are largely the same. Where the cleavage is beginning to appear is between that group of hospitals and the public hospitals. Public hospitals are beginning to drift apart as Ruth Hanft mentioned this morning. I think that is something that concerns us all.

Dr. Basil J. F. Mott: I accept that you and the other leaders in your organization and the others, as well, are genuinely motivated to provide the same quality of medical care that is associated with the voluntary sector.

My question is, to what extent does the existence of the voluntary sector help the decision-makers in investor-owned hospitals resist tendencies in the world of business that might work against the values that I know you and your colleagues share, such as inappropriate commercialization?

Dr. John H. Moxley III: Well, it is a very tough question for me to answer in a quantitative fashion. I was in the university system for a number of years, and I frequently get a question of "Haven't you noticed dramatic differences in the world you are in now. Isn't it 180 degrees different than what you were in before?" The answer to that is clearly no.

I detect no difference in goals and ideals in terms of the sorts of things that we are talking about in the senior managers at AMI than I did in the senior members of the faculty of the University of California, the University of Maryland, and Harvard Medical School. I just don't see it. Now, it could be that over the years, as you have pointed out, all hospitals and health care have been moving toward that sort of mentality and we are now just seeing a joining of it. But there was clearly no sharp difference when I stepped from one to the other.

Dr. Alonzo Yerby, *Director, Division of Health Services Administration, Uniformed Services University of Health Sciences*: A few years ago I had an opportunity to look at what passed for a quality-assurance program for one of the large chains, and it was ridiculous. It was a patient questionnaire that had little to do with quality. I hope that was an exception. I wonder what the status is of quality assurance in the organizations that you are involved with or indeed with the industry itself.

Dr. John H. Moxley III: Well, Al, the status is I think that all of the things that all hospitals do, including HCA, are worth about as much in one sector as in the other.

Beyond that, at a minimum of every other year, every one of our hospitals is visited by a team that is made up of a senior manager of the company, a medical record consultant, and a nurse. They go in and interview for two days physicians, people from the community, board members, and all the department heads in the hospital. Then they write a report that does receive a lot of scrutiny, and, although it is not quality of care in a sophisticated way they are critical, and they do initiate change.

Dr. Alonzo Yerby: Do they look at anything or do they just ask questions? Do they look at any records or rates?

Dr. John H. Moxley III: Well, rates are discussed at that time, but also at other times. They do look at some medical records. They are not clinical care experts that go through and try to analyze what the physician has done. They look at the records in terms of are they complete and up to date, etc. But I must say, again, without trying to be cynical, we did not do that at the University of California.

Ms. Ruth Hanft, *Consultant in Health Policy Research, Washington, D.C.*: I would like to pick up on what Bryan Luce said and also ask Dr. Mott something. I agree with Dr. Mott about the ideal, but I would like to ask him to respond in the context of the way physicians have behaved since the early 1900s and the whole concept of the fee-for-service system. The first for-profit hospitals were started by physicians, not by companies, and the growth and the development of the proprietary dialysis industry was basically physician-sponsored.

I think we have to distinguish between the voluntary religious and public hospitals as they evolved, and, as Professor Uwe Reinhardt of Princeton University so aptly calls it, the purveyors of medical care and the physicians. I think we have long had a dichotomy by calling it a nonprofit industry when the physician sector of the industry has always been a for-profit sector, and this kind of troubles me intellectually. Would you care to respond?

Dr. Basil J. F. Mott: First of all, I use the word profit differently. That someone is being paid a fee or a salary I don't think is a profit. I would rather use the word strictly as income that is distributed to stockholders who are owners; however, if physicians are in fact further identified as stockholders, then they are making a profit.

I think one of the problems that the voluntary hospitals have, maybe more so than the investor-owned, is that they have, in some respects, given in to a kind of entrepreneurism on the part of practitioners beyond what I think they really should be doing as community institutions.

I think there is something of a split personality in the nonprofit hospitals sector between the hospital as a community institution on the one hand governed by a group of lay citizens concerned about the welfare of the community, and, on the other hand, the hospital as a doctor's workshop in which individual physicians conduct private businesses called practices. However I do not see that problem being one that defeats the basic value system from which the voluntary hospital emerged, even though it is a long way from realizing the ideal.

Dr. John J. F. Moxley III: Dr. Mott, just to try to clarify: If a physician or a group of physicians are in practice and own the office building that they practice in, and they practice there all year, and then at the end of that year, they distribute the surplus among the practitioners in relationship to that which they brought in, and an individual practioner takes that sum and divides it up into individual trusts for his children or for whatever purposes, what would you call that bundle of money?

Dr. Basil J. F. Mott: Well, that's a profit. I personally, think that physicians at times are in a bind and seem to be changing their medical ethics. I think it is wrong if it's earned as a stockholder from a business if it is in a physician's economic interest to increase profits.

Dr. John H. Moxley III: What if he was a sole entrepreneur all by himself and happened to own the one room that he practiced in, and after paying the nurse and everything at the end of the year, had a bundle of money left over, and he took that money and again invested it or put it in his children's trust, what would you call that?

Dr. Basil J. F. Mott: The essence of what you are talking about is capitalism versus being paid for your services.

That someone is paid for their services does not make it a profit any more than I earn a profit because I am on salary, if I am following you correctly. I think the situation in which a physician owns an interest in a health enterprise in which he gains or may gain a benefit by referring patients or utilizing the services is in a conflict of interest that should be unacceptable.

Dr. John H. Moxley III: But the FAH data indicate that almost all physicians feel that way also. In fact, of the physicians that have ownership interests in hospitals, 79 percent or 80 percent of them have interest in hospitals that they have founded and started as individual proprietary hospitals. About 20 percent of physicians have owned stock in one of the large investor-owned companies.

Again, it is a potential conflict of interest, but in almost every case 60 to 70 percent of the stock of the investor-owned companies are held by institutional investors, trust funds, and pension funds, and so forth one could postulate the actual conflict of influencing that with research.

Mr. Jon Gabel, *Economist, National Center for Health Services Research*: I would like to raise an issue about quality of care. Once monetarization is acceptable in health care, then we are also saying that the market works. When the market works, consumers know what is best for them. If consumers know what is best for them, they can detect different levels in the quality of care. So why do we need occupational licensure?

Dr. James LoGerfo: The notion of the licensure basically sets an entry-level floor in the quality of inputs. It would be very difficult to be in that licensure system for anyone to establish a track record without a lot of murder and mayhem going on before consumers stumbled onto the fact that this was a poor provider of care, be that a physician, or a nurse practitioner, or anyone.

So the notion of licensure in the whole professional context is clearly as a social contract, something the public allows a profession to do. It sets a minimum floor on the entry-level input. There may be variation amongst the outputs in terms of their quality of care, no question about that, but at least it sets some minimum floor.

Mr. Jon Gabel: But I can tell the difference between a quack and a good practitioner more easily than I can tell the difference between nonprofit hospitals and for-profit hospitals.

Dr. James LoGerfo: I would agree with you that it is very difficult to distinguish the behavior of the for-profits and not-for-profits. There was a study on "dumping" to Southern California public hospital emergency rooms, and basically all of those patients that were sent to that emergency room came from not-for-profit institutions.

Ms. Helen Darling, *Director, Human Resources Studies, Government Research Corporation:* I am struck by the fact that a lot of the conversation is as if there were truly shrinking resources in the total dollars in health care, and I know they are not shrinking, but they are growing dramatically.

Secondly, everybody wants their piece of the pie, and the number who want that piece is growing. One of the reasons that everybody is in trouble financially is that there are too many hospitals, too many people functioning at inefficient levels.

One could actually argue that what is happening, even with its problems and with the danger to quality, actually forces some closing in a way that the old charitable system never gave us, even though a lot of people tried to find out where the federal and local dollars went. But I am intrigued that nobody talked about how many of the problems that we have in terms of resources and quality relate to what has been an increasingly worsening problem of excess capacity in the institutional end.

Dr. Basil J. F. Mott: I think we are sitting around this table not because the health care system has been a dismal failure, but because it has been so successful, because the American public is so enamored of medicine. The problem is that we have a discontinuity with our ability economically to satisfy these expectations.

We all agree that we probably have the best system in the world. Our problem is that our expectations are rising and becoming an increasing financial burden. We put in place with Medicare and Medicaid a system of payment which has given everybody bad habits and encouraged the worst kind of utilization of resources. We see the terrible scandals happening in the defense industry because cost-plus contracting. I just think we ought to be clear that we have a good thing going, it is just that we have a problem in satisfying expectations and dealing with resources, or would you disagree on that?

Ms. Helen Darling: I do not disagree.

Mr. Myles Lash, *formerly Executive Director of Hospital Administration, Medical College of Virginia, Richmond, VA; currently, National Director of Health Care, Arthur Young and Company*: I was interested sometime back on the quick answer relative to advertisement. It seems to me if organizations are developing quality parameters, and they can be objectively understood by the public, then why shouldn't hospitals acknowledge these standards and their respective performance through the media? I can remember the debate five years ago over the appropriateness of hospital advertising, but in many states all sorts of health care advertising exists, all the barriers have been eliminated by the competitive market place. Although it often makes us uncomfortable, I do not think the public would suffer listening to some objective information rather than the heavenly hymns I am now hearing on TV.

Dr. John H. Moxley III: Anyone who has been to Minneapolis-St. Paul recently will know that health care institutions are advertising and doing so intensively. You cannot watch TV for more than 15 minutes without seeing a few advertisements. I still find that bothersome.

Mr. John Ryan, *President, Ryan Advisors, Inc.*: I would like to comment on what Dr. Mott just said. If we had been doing in the airline industry what we did in the health industry, allowing people access to planes relatively inexpensively, then the Mayo Clinic would not be expanding into Jacksonville and Phoenix, but instead Rochester Minnesota Airport would have to be expanding.

Dr. John H. Moxley III: We have a subsidiary alternative service company that is called Diagnostic Services, Inc., which is a mobile CAT scanning company. It has CAT scanners that service more than one hospital. Before going into that business, the parameters that we established were that we would not proceed unless we could operate efficiently and effectively, with the same quality that one would find in a hospital.

We have maintained that standard. The company is concerned with improving the imaging capability of the hospitals that it serves and not competing with them. Mobile CAT scanning capability is brought to the hospital on a regular basis, as well as on an emergency basis.

Mr. John Ryan: I also have a question for Dr. Moxley. It is my understanding that as the Alternative Services Director, you are developing up to 75 free-standing imaging departments throughout the country. How is that program going to impact your own hospital as well as other hospitals?

Dr. John H. Moxley III: We are, at the present time, looking at free-standing imaging centers. We have only one that is under construction; that is at University of California at Irvine. It is a joint venture with the University of California to determine how a free-standing imaging center structured around MRI is going to perform in relation to the hospital, in relation to the faculty, and so forth. It is in the research and development phase at the present time. If it is successful, then we may well market the concept elsewhere.

There have been a number of large group practices who have been anxious to talk about it, because it is something they want to add to their capability as a large multispecialty practice. It is in the development stage, which is not to say we might not end up having 75 or 200.

Mr. Samuel Mitchell, *Director of Research, Federation of American Hospitals*: Dr. Mott has drawn a distinction between commercial values and health care values; I think that the distinction has been overdone. The for-profit hospital exists only for one reason – that is to please customers or patients. Intentions count only insofar as they lead to desirable results. We do not survive unless we make patients well, if we can. So the problem is not that there is a dichotomy in values; the problem is that some people do not have the money to command the market's attention, namely indigents. And teaching and research are indeed public goods.

The solution is to enfranchise people who currently are not enfranchised by somehow subsidizing them.

In short, the dichotomy comes on the demand side in that some people in society do not have the wherewithal to get adequate care. We all have an obligation, investor-owneds included, to make sure that access to adequate care is universal. That is a very separate issue from for-profits.

Dr. Basil J. F. Mott: I may very well be overdrawing the value of that, but I believe that there is a conflict here, and you put your finger right on it discussing the patient as a customer. It seems to me you are putting the patient in a role which I think leaves out something very fundamental. A patient is someone who has given him or herself up to someone who is called a professional in whom the individual must trust that he or she is going to be treated with a degree of altruism and a concern for his or her welfare that goes beyond any corporate, organizational, or institutional values.

There is even a conflict between altruism and self interest within the voluntary hospital. I believe that when we turn to a physician or other caregivers (the physician is the key person in this), we are turning to someone whom we regard as engaged, at least in part in a calling, and who does not view us in the way the word "customer" is normally used in our society, which comes essentially from the business world.

There is something of an intrinsic value in caring for people who are ill that cannot be encompassed within the concept of customer. Probably there is not time to unfold this issue here, but I think that is where a number of the problems are located.

Dr. Steve Eastaugh, *Associate Professor, Department of Health Services Administration, The George Washington University.*: I have two quick points to make following up on Sam Mitchell's question and also Bryan Luce's question about arrogance. It seems to me that in some sense it is a good thing that the investor-owned sector is pressuring us, in the nonprofit sector, at least, to get rid of our arrogance and to develop some acumen as far as business management mentality. What can improve the efficiency of the sector is the three-legged stool concept that works for Japanese business:

(1) quality control, (2) marketing, and (3) productivity. The investor-owneds have been doing a good job of pressuring us in those areas.

To follow up on Sam's point, I encountered an example of marketing in the investor-owned sector doing good things when I visited an investor-owned hospital in Florida. As I am from the Northeast, I am not too familiar with investor-owneds, and I visited this particular investor-owned hospital where they have completed a survey of women's preferences concerning such things as birthing centers and other maternity care alternatives. They were not interested in health promotion; they were interested in bringing in revenues, needless to say. But the hospital offered an alternative, and it sold quite well. One thing I think investor-owneds do very well compared to, say, tax-exempt gentlemen's clubs such as Mass. General, is they do not have an arrogance about marketing. Marketing is simply doing right by the patient: determining what consumers require and tailoring services to meet those needs.

They believe there are two kinds of customers in a hospital and vis-a-vis hospital health services, if you will. One set of customers are the physicians, but another new active articulate customer is the patient. Investor-owned facilities go out and do preference surveys of patients, marketing analyses, and conjoint measurement techniques. If you think marketing is simply selling and advertising, you have never taken a business course in marketing. Marketing is getting out and finding what the patient, the ultimate customer, really wants.

I do not have time to say anything more about quality control or productivity, but I think pressuring us as non-profits to perform a little better, is a good thing.

I do want to make one last quick point, though, about the poor. There is an idea that perhaps investor-owneds shunned the poor, and we should endow unfunded care. I am all for endowing unfunded care, and with sufficient funding to last in perpetuity. There is a national problem with uncompensated care. I feel that just because investor-owned setup offers the incentives, if you will, a window of opportunity to cut back on care does not mean that professionals necessarily avail themselves of those opportunities.

I visited, within the last few months, investor-owned and voluntaries in Louisiana and in Florida. Unlike Massachusetts where there is no clear dichotomy among hospitals, the Southern nonpublic hospitals are doing 3–8 percent uncompensated care and the public hospitals are doing 80–99 percent. I believe if you examine the statistics you will see that if you compare the voluntary sector in a given neighborhood in the south of the Sunbelt to an investor-owned, nonpublic hospitals are both doing a very small amount of uncompensated care. Most of the uncompensated care is done in hospitals in terrible shape as far as the plant and equipment are concerned, as in the Charity Hospital in New Orleans.

So, I really think that this idea that the investor-owneds are shunning the poor just is not so. You should not quote the *New England Journal of Medicine* or statistics elsewhere comparing the nonprofits in Boston to investor-owneds in the south and the Sunbelt and assume that it means that the south and the Sunbelt must be cream skimming the investor-owneds down there. The voluntaries are cream skimming and avoiding and dumping, if you will, just as much as the investor-owneds are. If hospitals more effectively select the right department to specialize in, so that they remain financially healthy, they can avoid picking and choosing between poor and well-insured patients.

Dr. Cecil Sheps, *Taylor Grandy Distinguished Professor of Social Medicine, The University of North Carolina at Chapel Hill:* I would like to make two comments. First, I have the impression that a good portion of the profitability for investor-owned hospital chains have until now come, not from the operation of the hospitals, but from their real estate operations, from their depreciation and other federal tax benefits which represent an expense to the general public. There has not been great pressure in the institution to be economic. The studies that compare the operational revenue of comparable institutions, investor-owned and non-profit, indicate that there is no significant difference. When we think about the future, we have to think about a different kind of future, as Dick Egdahl mentioned. I think we can see indications that that is going to change, so the pressure might be different.

Secondly, on the question of customer satisfaction and customer security, I think they are not the same, though there has been some progress in this regard since the days when I was a hospital administrator in Boston. I want to tell you that, after a year or two there, I began to say to my colleagues, "If you want your hospital to have a good reputation, there are two things you need. It is good that the coffee is hot and so on, but it helps to have an obstetrical service, because somehow people tend to give the hospital credit for that beautiful baby. The second thing is, when patients die, whether the death was preventable or not, to be certain that everyone comforts the family and helps them deal with their sense of grief.

You have then established a good reputation." I have checked this with other people, and they indicate that I am right.

Finally, on the question of customer security as opposed to customer satisfaction, I am constantly plagued by the fact that for years the automobile manufacturers in this country were selling automobiles that they knew were grossly defective and dangerous. It was not until Ralph Nader published his book on the subject and drew public attention to it that we developed much more accountability on this issue. I would like to be assured that this experience is not typical of what is likely to happen when hospitals are operated, in the last analysis, to return profits to the investors and, if at all possible, more each year.

Access

WARREN GREENBERG, PH.D.
Associate Professor,
Department of Health Services Administration,
The George Washington University,
Washington, D.C.

Introductory Remarks: Access to Health Care

Economists assume that for-profit hospitals attempt to maximize profits and that non-profit hospitals attempt to achieve a net income equal to or greater than zero. In addition, non-profit hospitals may have other objectives such as accumulating sophisticated technology; increasing market share; or even maximizing physician income (Pauly and Redisch, 1973). It has also been suggested that non-profits may have altruistic objectives such as providing care to indigent individuals (Relman, 1980). Whatever the objectives of a non-profit hospital, the important point is that it faces a financial constraint.

When a non-profit hospital may potentially realize a negative net income because of increased competition or regulation, non-profit hospitals may curtail objectives in which costs exceed benefits. Such objectives may include accepting indigent patients or patients for whom the costs of treatment exceed reimbursement rates.

Under cost-based reimbursement, where a hospital is virtually certain of breaking even, one might expect to find non-profit hospitals pursuing some avenues, such as accepting indigent patients, which may not be cost effective. In contrast, under constraints on reimbursement or under increased competition from other hospitals, access to the non-profits, like the for-profit hospitals, may be based on a hospital's benefit-cost calculation.

An example from the health insurance industry which includes the non-profit Blue Cross firms as well as the for-profit commercial carriers may illustrate the behavior of non-profit firms in the hospital industry.

Professor Philip Fanara and I found in a recent study that Blue Cross, when confronted with increased competition from health maintenance organizations (HMOs), and when regulated by state insurance commissions, enrolled a decreased proportion of higher-risk, non-group individuals (Fanara and Greenberg, 1985). Non-group individuals usually have hospital utilization rates markedly higher than individuals who are members of a group insurance plan.

Without increased competition and regulation, Blue Cross plans accepted a greater proportion of non-group enrollees. Confronted with a potential reduction in net income, Blue Cross behavior approached that of the for-profit commercial carriers, which under any competitive or regulatory climate, do not have incentives to enroll individuals in which costs would exceed income.

Since the late 1970s there have been increasing restraints on the reimbursement of hospitals as well as other providers. Many state governments have initiated mandatory prospective reimbursement programs in response to rising health care costs. Other states have used competitive bidding among hospitals as a way to contain costs. In the private sector, insurers have also utilized prospective reimbursement as well as utilization review. The federal government began reimbursing hospitals on a diagnosis-related-group (DRG) basis for Medicare enrollees in October 1983.

In summary, therefore, I would expect with constraints on reimbursement as well as increased competition, to observe similar behavior of for-profit and non-profit institutions – restricting access to indigent patients and to patients in which the costs of treatment exceed reimbursement rates. A market failure exists here in which government intervention appears to be necessary.

In the hospital sector, both Vraciu and Shortell suggest that there is little evidence to support the proposition that non-profit and for-profit hospitals differ in their relative accessibility of health care services, although Shortell cites recent state evidence by the Institute of Medicine which suggests that for-profit hospitals may treat relatively fewer indigent patients. Large differences appear, however, between for-profit and non-profit hospitals on one hand and public hospitals, which have taken a greater number of low-income individuals, on the other. Both authors suggest that access to all hospitals is an important health financing concern that must be addressed by public policy officials.

Two important points should be made about the Vraciu and Shortell contributions on access. First, access is measured, in part, in the studies referenced by Vraciu and Shortell, by percentage of Medicare and Medicaid patients or percent of indigents in non-profit and for-profit hospitals in particular states and areas. Yet, in many states and areas, there are very few or no for-profit hospitals. This may be due to excessive regulation in these states and areas which serve to keep out for-profit firms, or to a reluctance of the for-profit firms to serve states and areas where there is low income population. If the latter explanation is in fact the case, the results of additional studies should reflect this point.

Second, each of the studies which have been examined by Vraciu and Shortell have used data prior to the advent of the DRG, prospective payment system in October 1983. Studies which examine the relative access of the for-profit and non-profit hospitals using data from the post-DRG period, might suggest an increasing propensity of both non-profit and for-profit hospitals to avoid costly patients.

It is possible that access to hospitals by the very sick and low-income groups may not be solved by restraining or limiting the growth of for-profit hospitals, but rather must be solved by public policy initiatives. This should not be viewed as an unusal proposition since, for example, the United States has not attempted to alleviate hunger among the poor by creating non-profit food establishments and food markets, but rather by providing food stamps to the indigent. Similarly, there have been no attempts to creat non-profit construction firms to supply housing and rental units to the poor. Subsidized housing and housing units, to at least some extent, have been made available to the poor. Even in the health care industry itself, there has been, perhaps surprisingly, virtually no suggestion that physician services, pharmaceuticals, technological equipment, dentists, or the majority of nursing homes be turned into non-profit institutions. In fact, one can sometimes wonder why it is necessarily the hospital which appears in the spotlight of the for-profit, non-profit controversy. It is true that the hospital accounts for forty percent of health care expenditures in the United States (the largest share of any aspect of the sector), but for example, physicians, although they only account for twenty percent of expenditures, are responsible for about seventy percent of health care costs.

REFERENCES

Pauly, Mark and Redisch, Michael. "The Not-for Profit Hospital as a Physicians' Cooperative." *American Economic Review*, 63(1):87–99, March 1973.

Relman, Arnold S. "The New Medical-Industrial Complex." *The New England Journal of Medicine*, 303(17):963–970, October 23, 1980.

Fanara, Philip Jr. and Greenberg, Warren. "The Impact of Competition and Regulation on Blue Cross Enrollment of Non-Group Individuals." *Journal of Risk and Insurance*, 211(2):185–198, June 1985.

ROBERT A. VRACIU, PH.D.
President, The Center for Health Studies, Hospital Corporation of America

PHYLLIS M. VIRGIL, M.P.A.
Manager, Strategic Planning, Hospital Corporation of America

The Impact of Investor Owned Hospitals on Access to Health Care

The rapid growth and financial success of large investor-owned hospital companies, such as the Hospital Corporation of America (HCA), has stimulated a new round of debate about investor-owned hospitals and the implications for the health care system. Arnold Relman (1980) perhaps stimulated this most recent round of debate with his article on the new medical-industrial complex.

Absent from much of this debate are the factual underpinnings of the behavior of *investor-owned hospitals* and a recognition that the term investor-owned hospital represents a very diverse group of autonomous corporations. Much of the controversy also fails to focus on the broader economic and organizational phenomena that are driving the health delivery system, including, but not limited to, investor-owned hospitals. Rather, discussion tends to focus on issues from a "good guy/bad guy" perspective, as if investor-owned hospital managers are driven by the simplest of economic motives – profit maximization. As we all learned in Economics 1A, the model described by Adam Smith is a useful pedagogic model, but nobody is really expected to behave that way. We went on to learn in Economics 2A, that in reality, large corporations go to great lengths to balance business imperatives with social responsibility.

Norman Mailer perhaps best captured the reason why we frequently perceive an issue through a narrow focus ". . . to the extent we invest in a particular scenario, we can always find ongoing evidence to keep living with it." As all actors in the health services industry place greater attention on the business aspects of their endeavors, a "good guy/bad guy" scenario will certainly find evidence, and perhaps reason, to place blame. Unfortunately, the "blame or credit" is likely to be attributed based on spurious correlation.

Contemporary issues, such as access to health care, are broad and complex enough that it would be very difficult, if not impossible, to isolate the independent impact of the growth of investor-owned hospitals on access. Consequently, our effort here is more modest in its attempt. First, we argue that access cannot be measured directly. Rather, we must limit our measurement to related indicators. Second, we describe investor-owned hospital behavior by studying illustrations of specific approaches or initiatives and by statistical comparisons with not-for-profit and/or government hospitals. Third, we briefly explore the "access issue" from a broader perspective, arguing that solutions to existing problems or ways to prevent future problems lie in societal/governmental actions, not in placing responsibility solely on the hospital industry.

FRAMEWORK FOR OBSERVATIONS

The concept of access to health care is complex. It has dimensions that go beyond the mere presence or availability of a resource in a given place at a given time. The data and observations presented in this paper deal with investor-owned hospitals as they relate to dimensions of access. To provide a framework for analysis, we view access in two ways: those factors or indicators that relate to availability of services and those that relate to accessibility. Table 1 illustrates the framework that we use to structure our discussion on the impact of ownership on access to health care.

We can define availability as a measure (in terms of type, volume, and location) of the supply of health resources and services relative to the needs or demands of a given individual or community. Health care is available to an individual when he can obtain it at the time and place that he needs it and from appropriate personnel (Subcommittee on Health, 1976). As shown in Table 1, our framework deals with availability in three ways:

1. **Hospital Operations** – the impact of investor-owned companies on the continued viability of community hospitals
2. **Service Mix** – differences among ownership type regarding

TABLE 1
FRAMEWORK FOR OBSERVATIONS
Comparisons with Investor-Owned Hospital Behavior

Area	Absence of Investor-Owned Hospitals	Other Hospital Providers	Norms or Expectations
Availability			
Hospital Operation	X		
Service Mix		X	
Physician Mix		X	
Accessibility			
Patient Mix		X	
Funding Sources	X		
Obligation Contracts	X		

the number and sophistication of services offered to a community

3. **Physician Mix** – variations in the number and type of physicians by ownership type

Accessibility can be defined as the ability of an individual or group to obtain medical care. Access has geographical, financial, social, ethical, and psychic components and is thus very difficult to define and measure operationally (Subcommittee on Health, 1976). To analyze availability, our framework deals with the following components of the concept:

1. **Patient Mix** – comparisons of the type of patient served by ownership status (this provides an outcome-based measure on whether disadvantaged patients are being served to the same degree)
2. **Funding Sources** – the involvement of investor-owned companies in creating a pool of funds to finance health services for the disadvantaged (funding pools generally arise in the transfer of ownership)

3. **Obligation Contracts** – the development of sales agreements that include explicit contractual obligations to provide care for the poor.

Our framework is divided into three types of comparisons. The first refers to what would have happened in the absence of investor-owned hospitals or an initiative by an investor-owned hospital company. It suggests that certain actions have made a difference in what would otherwise have been a default situation. The second type of comparison shows actions of investor-owned hospitals relative to other hospital providers. For example, do investor-owned hospitals have the same service mix as not-for-profit hospitals? The question of whether behavior patterns are appropriate for either group is not addressed. The third column represents comparisons that can lead to good versus bad judgments. Due to a lack of data, we have not focused on comparisons of investor-owned hospitals (or any hospital, for that matter). In addition, there remain many unanswered questions that relate to access, including:

- What should hospitals offer?
- Who should have what kind of access to available hospital services?
- Will there be equality of access?
- How will service for the disadvantaged be financed?

Consequently, our ability is limited in this paper to assess what is occuring in the hospital industry as it relates to the complex question of access. Access is measured in terms of related observations of behavior, and assessments are limited to investor-owned contributions relative to not-for-profit and government facilities (in some cases). The absence of widely accepted standards precludes much discussion at this point about the good versus bad of observable behavior.

AVAILABILITY – HOSPITAL OPERATIONS

Investor-owned hospital companies often come to communities because of problems associated with existing not-for-profit and government facilities. Frequently, such hospitals are in poor financial condition and are facing major property, plant, and equipment expenditures. The access question relates to whether access would be better if the hospital went out of business or continued to operate on an undercapitalized basis?

While investor-owned hospital companies are not the only source of capital and management talent for financially distressed hospitals, they are the ones aggressively seeking to acquire or lease community hospitals. The benefits brought to many communities by investor-owned companies include:

1. **Access to Capital** – Over the next ten years, it is estimated that at least $125 billion in capital will be needed to replace or remodel Hill-Burton hospitals (Shaw, 1984). Relying heavily on debt financing, many not-for-profits will likely face severe capital constraints as sources of debt financing become increasingly scarce. Compared to the not-for-profit industry, investor-owned systems are well positioned to secure future capital funds by tapping both debt and equity markets. Affiliation with the investor-owned sector, then, may be one of few options for those not-for-profits that face pressing capital needs.
2. **Highly Qualified Management Talent** – Given the size, importance, or status of many community hospitals, investor-owned companies can often place better management talent than a community could hope to attract. In addition, the functional specialists found at many of the large investor-owned systems can bring to community hospitals specialized expertise that otherwise would not be available.
3. **Financial Stability** – As with many new undertakings, hospitals acquired by investor-owned companies must frequently be subsidized for a period of time before they are financially stable. Thus, the investor-owned sector can draw its system-wide resources to cross-subsidize hospitals that would otherwise face closure or operate under substandard conditions.
4. **Health Care Professionals** – By using national recruiting networks, large systems can find and place needed health care professionals. This is especially advantageous in single-hospital communities, where the health care professional is commonly a scarce resource.

These are just some examples of what investor-owned companies can bring to a community. Specific impact, however, will vary from community to community.

AVAILABILITY– SERVICE MIX

To date, there is no national consensus on the appropriate scope and mix of health services for a community. Nevertheless, the number and sophistication of services made available to a consumer affect community access to services.

It has been argued that investor-owned hospitals provide fewer services than voluntary hospitals and thus do not address the population's need for access to a broad range of services. The question relating to service mix is the "allegation" that investor-owned hospitals selectively provide services based on profitability rather than community need. It should be noted that profitability is a relative term and that it is not possible to state clearly which services are profitable and which are unprofitable. For example, obstetrics is frequently thought of as a loss leader. However, if a facility's obstetrics volume is high, the service will probably generate profits. Likewise, high-technology services can be either winners or losers depending on the volume of services a hospital is able to generate.

Using available evidence, we can determine if service mix variations do exist between ownership types. These measurements of service mix can provide some answers to the following questions:

- Does the number of services considered basic and essential to a community vary according to ownership?
- Does the scope of services or the total number of inpatient services available at a hospital differ among ownership types?
- Is service sophistication and willingness to offer unprofitable service different in investor-owned hospitals than in not-for-profit hospitals?

Basic Services

It has been argued that investor-owned hospitals may not ensure the availability of services considered basic and essential to a community, particularly if doing so is not profitable. The question relating to access is, Does ownership type significantly affect the number of basic services offered? To explore this issue we used the **Basic** services measure of Ralph E. Berry, Jr., (1973) who defines **Basic** as those services most hospitals offer: clinical laboratory, emergency room, operating room, delivery room, and diagnostic x-ray. Information on hospital ownership, size, and services for all nonfederal , short-term, general medical/surgical hospitals was obtained from the 1980 American Hospital Association (AHA) data files. Four states – Florida, Tennessee, Texas, and California – were selected for the study due to their high percentages of investor-owned chain hospitals.

To determine the impact of ownership on basic services, ordinary least squares regression was performed. The study grouped hospitals by ownership into four categories: (1) state, district, or county hospitals (public); (2) not-for-profit hospitals (voluntary); (3) investor-owned chain hospitals (IOC); and (4) freestanding, investor-owned hospitals (FIO). Other independent variables are included in the analysis to control for effects that may mask the unique impact of **Ownership** on **Basic** services:

- **Bedtotal** – hospital size as measured by the total number of beds set up and staffed
- **Metro** – the hospital's location in either an urban or rural area
- **Bedshare** – the competitive position of a hospital with others in the area as measured by the proportion of beds within a county owned by a given hospital.

Table 2 presents the results for the basic services variable as affected by **Ownership** and **Bedshare**. Our basic variable consisted of four services originally classified by Berry as basic; the fifth, diagnostic x-ray, was not included as a distinct category in AHA's 1980 Annual Survey. Since the range of the basic variable is from 0 to 4 (a value of 4 indicates that a hospital has all four basic services), the averages of 3–3.5 indicate that most basic services are available.

Comparing voluntary with investor-owned system hospitals, we find that the range of basic services offered is similar between ownership type. The findings also show that the average number of basic

TABLE 2
Number of Basic Services by County Bedshare and Ownership Non-Federal Short-Term General Hospitals

Regression Results*				
Public	Voluntary	Investor Owned Chains	Freestanding Investor-Owned	Bedshare in %
3.4	3.3	3.1	3.2	10
3.4	3.4	3.2	3.3	25
3.4	3.5	3.3	3.3	60
3.5	3.6	3.5	3.3	90

*See Appendix A for regression coefficients and levels of significance.

services increases as a hospital's share of total community beds increases, that both types of hospitals offer fewer basic services in counties in which there are many hospitals, and that in those counties for which there is only one primary provider, both ownership types provide virtually identical numbers of basic services. These results indicate that basic services are perceived to be basic to communities rather than to individual hospitals. Further analysis found that in non-metropolitan areas, there appears to be an equal commitment by investor-owned system hospitals and voluntary hospitals to provide the community with a range of essential needs.

Service Scope

Using the same data base and independent variables as in the **Basic** service analysis, we went on to explore differences in total service (**Servtot**), or the number of inpatient services available at a hospital, among ownership types. This analysis also uses ordinary least squares regression to determine the impact of the independent variables – **Ownership**, **Bedtotal**, and **Metro** – on the dependent variable **Servtot**. As Table 3 below shows, when grouped by bed size, there appears to be little difference in the total number

TABLE 3
Expected Total Number of Services (Servtot)
by Bed Size and Ownership
Non-Federal Short-Term General Hospitals

Regression Results*

Public	Voluntary	Investor-Owned Chains	Freestanding Investor-Owned Hospitals	Bedtotal
18.9	18.2	19.7	16.6	50
25.8	25.1	24.9	23.4	150
31.7	30.9	29.0	29.3	250
36.5	35.8	32.1	34.1	350

*See Appendix for regression coefficients and levels of significance.

of services offered between voluntary and investor-owned company hospitals. In fact, bed size explained almost 65 percent of the variation in the scope of services offered.

The above estimates also indicate that small investor-owned system hospitals are likely to have more services, while large investor-owned system hospitals are likely to have fewer services than other hospital types. This suggests that small investor-owned system hospitals appear to be providing a broader range of services than other hospital types. Furthermore, voluntary hospitals seem to provide relatively fewer services in metropolitan areas and relatively more in non-metropolitan areas. The narrowing of service scope, however, may be due to rational economic responses to competitive environments where some specialization is likely to occur.

Service Sophistication and Profitability

Another common belief is that investor-owned hospitals avoid offering services that lose money, leaving the not-for-profit hospitals to provide them. To address this issue, a recent study by Frank A. Sloan and Robert A. Vraciu (1983) compared the services available at not-for-profit hospitals with those offered by investor-owned hospitals in Florida.

Florida was selected for several reasons. First, comparable data were available for analysis. Second, Florida's large investor-owned industry provided an adequate sample for valid comparisons. Using 1980 data from the AHA Annual Survey, the study compared non-federal, short-term general, non-teaching hospitals under 400 beds. This category contained the vast majority of Florida's community hospitals. Table 4 summarizes the study's results.

These results show that investor-owned system hospitals in Florida provided a larger percentage of emergency services (80 percent) than did the not-for-profit hospitals (72.5 percent). The data tend to refute the argument that investor-owned hospitals do not offer outpatient or emergency services because they are so often used by people unable to pay. The two ownership types also were comparable in offering radiology, laboratory, and pharmacy capabilities, those services considered "profitable" under charge-based reimbursement. Furthermore, the not-for-profits were more likely to offer profitable services, such as open heart surgery, cardiac catheterization, and computerized axial tomography scanning, and unprofitable services like premature nursery. In summary, except for cardiac care, this study suggests that not-for-profits and

TABLE 4
Florida Facilities and Services, 1981

Facility or Service	Type of Hospital, in %: Nonprofit	Investor-Owned: Total	Investor-Owned: Systems
Postoperative Recovery Room	90.2	83.1	88.9
Pharmacy with Registered Pharmacist: Full-time	84.2	83.0	88.9
Pharmacy with Registered Pharmacist: Part-time	7.8	1.7	2.2
Histopathology Laboratory	76.5	72.9	77.8
Electroencephalography	86.3	79.7	86.7
Respiratory Therapy Services	92.5	83.1	88.9
Physical Therapy Services	90.2	83.0	91.1
Occupational Therapy Services	23.1	30.5	31.1
Dental Services	56.8	33.9	40.0
Podiatric Services	45.1	44.1	53.3
Speech Pathology Services	39.2	40.7	40.0
Volunteer Services Department	58.8	61.0	64.4
Patient Representative Services	56.9	44.1	51.1
Social Work Services	86.3	76.3	82.2
Hospital Auxiliary	78.4	37.6	64.4
Premature Nursery	29.4	5.1	6.7
Abortion Services (Inpatient)	31.4	32.2	33.3
Abortion Services (Outpatient)	11.8	16.9	20.0
Hospice	2.0	3.4	4.4
Emergency Department	72.5	71.2	80.0
Organized Outpatient Department	43.1	32.2	40.0
Rehabilitation Outpatient Services	17.6	11.9	15.6
Organ Bank	0.0	1.7	2.2
Blood Bank	60.8	69.4	73.3
Genetic Counseling Services	0.0	0.0	0.0
Open-Heart Surgery Facilities	13.7	6.8	8.9
Alcoholism/Chemical Dependency Outpatient Services	7.8	3.4	4.4

Psychiatric Services			
Emergency	21.6	11.9	15.6
Outpatient	9.8	5.1	6.7
Partial Hospitalization	9.8	1.7	0.0
Foster and/or Home Care	0.0	0.0	0.0
Consultation and Education	23.5	13.6	15.6
Clinical Psychology Services	9.8	10.2	13.3
Radiation Therapy			
X-ray	13.7	11.9	15.6
Megavoltage	11.8	5.1	6.7
Radioactive Implants	27.5	15.3	17.8
Radioisotope Facilities			
Diagnostic	80.3	76.3	60.0
Therapeutic	19.6	13.6	13.3
Family Planning Services	2.0	0.0	0.0
Home Care Department	7.8	3.4	2.2
Computerized Axial Tomography	39.2	27.1	24.4
Cardiac Catheterization	15.7	6.8	8.9
Number of Hospitals in Data Base	52	60	45

*Adapted from Frank A. Sloan and Robert A. Vraciu. "Investor-Owned and Not-For-Profit Hospitals: Addressing Some Issues." *Health Affairs*, 2 (1), Spring 1983, 25–37.

investor-owned system hospitals are comparable, both in terms of service sophistication and willingness to provide unprofitable services.

On the whole, the data on service mix suggests that the behavior of investor-owned hospitals and not-for-profit hospitals is similar. However, judgments regarding service mix variations are difficult since more or fewer services may be good or bad depending on circumstances. For example, what impact does service mix patterns have on duplication of services or on competition? The answer will vary according to policy initiatives and desired outcomes.

AVAILABILITY–PHYSICIAN SERVICES

There are a number of cases where investor-owned hospital companies have acquired county or not-for-profit hospitals and improved the medical staff complement. The Stones River Hospital case

(Woodbury versus Tennessee) illustrates one such case. Following acquisition and replacement of an existing hospital, the hospital was able to attract and retain specialists that could not be recruited previously. Having specialties such as orthopedics, dermatology, rheumatology, and neurology available within the community improved access in a geographic sense because it reduced the need for referrals to hospitals outside of town. (Bryant, 1984)

On a broader basis, investor-owned and not-for-profit hospitals have medical staffs of similar sizes and primary/specialty mixes. Analysis of the medical staff information on the 1982 AHA Hospital Survey Tapes support this conclusion when statistically analyzed for the number of primary, specialty, and total physicians on the medical staff, while controlling for community size and average daily census, the ownership variables had virtually identical independent impacts.

ACCESSIBILITY– PATIENT MIX

The question addressed by patient mix is whether ownership status has an impact on access to services for those groups unable to pay the full hospital bill. A review of patients paying less than charges (i.e., Medicare, Medicaid, and indigent patients) sheds some light on hospital behavior.

Medicare and Medicaid

It is well known that Medicare and Medicaid reimburse at less than full hospital charges. Medicare reimbursements are approximately 30 percent less than charges, (Health Care Financing Review, 1982) and Medicaid payments are frequently less than actual cost of providing services. In 1981, the total payment shortfall from Medicare and Medicaid amounted to $4.8 billion (Southeastern Hospital Conference, 1983). While providing services to these groups of patients will likely benefit a hospital financially, reimbursement will be less than what a facility would otherwise receive from privately insured populations.

Evidence suggests that the behavior patterns of both investor-owned and not-for-profit are relatively similar in the amount of care provided to Medicare and Medicaid patients. In fact, several studies show investor-owned hospitals as providing a higher percentage of care to one or both patient groups.

One study of hospitals in Florida found that in 1980 there were no meaningful differences between not-for-profit and investor-owned hospitals. Compared with investor-owned hospitals, the not-for-profits were slightly lower in the percentage of total patient days provided to Medicare patients (57 percent for not-for-profits versus 58.5 percent for investor-owned) and Medicaid patients (2.9 percent and 4.2 percent respectively) (Sloan and Vraciu, 1983). In 1981, similar patterns of care occurred in Florida. Again, there were no significant differences between ownership types (State of Florida, 1983).

Comparing not-for-profit hospitals with investor-owned system hospitals, Lewin and Associates (Lewin, Derzon, and Margulies, 1983) found similar behavior patterns in its study of hospitals in California, Florida, and Texas. Using 1978 data, the percentage of Medicare days provided was 45 percent for investor-owned hospitals versus 47 percent for not-for-profits; both ownership types provided 8 percent of total patient days to Medicaid patients.

Evidence also suggests that hospital system behavior is comparable among ownership type. One study of major multi-hospital systems (Bernstein, 1983) found that in 1982 relatively similar amounts of care were delivered to Medicare and Medicaid patients regardless of ownership status. As a percentage of gross revenue, the investor-owned company hospitals cared for a larger percentage of Medicare and Medicaid patients (50 percent) than the average for all hospital systems (45 percent).

It should also be noted that although Medicaid service levels are equal for not-for-profit and investor-owned hospitals, public hospitals provide significantly more care to Medicaid patients. In Florida, for example, government hospitals provided 8.3 percent of total patient days to Medicaid patients in 1982, compared with 4.9 percent for all hospitals (State of Florida Cost Containment Board, 1984). While this figure is high, it is not surprising, since the primary mission of public hospitals is to provide care for those unable to pay.

Uncompensated Care

Few would deny that hospitals should share the burdens created by financially disadvantaged patients. However, until a consensus is reached on how to finance care for those that cannot pay, there is no standard to measure whether hospitals have met their obligation. The only empirical approach is to measure relative behavior of investor-owned and not-for-profit hospitals. We measure a hospital's burden in terms of the amount of uncompensated care (i.e., the sum of allowances for charity and bad debts). Separating the two is meaningless because of variations in accounting practices.

As with the amount of care provided to Medicare and Medicaid patients, ownership status does not appear to impact access for those unable to pay. An investigation of Florida hospitals in 1980 found that on a per patient day basis, ownership groups have virtually identical uncompensated care loads. Both not-for-profit hospitals and total investor-owned hospitals offset revenues $16, and investor-owned hospital systems offset revenues $15 per patient day for uncompensated care. This suggests that in Florida, investor-owned and not-for-profit hospitals treat indigent patients similarly (Sloan and Vraciu, 1983). Comparing multi-hospital systems, another study also found that investor-owned company hospitals provide about the same amount of free care (3.3 percent of all patients served) as all multi-hospital systems and all hospitals nationally–3.3 percent and 3.5 percent, respectively (Bernstein and Co., 1983).

Differential performance in providing uncompensated care on a broader basis can be investigated by looking at data on 2,260 hospitals obtained from the 1982 AHA Annual Survey. Figure 1 shows uncompensated care as a percentage of charges by hospital ownership, location, and bed size.

With the uncompensated care percentage as the dependent variable, regression analysis enables us to answer the following questions: Are differences among hospital types statistically significant? Does the relationship among teaching, ownership, and the dependent variable disappear when other factors, such as bed size, facility mix, payer mix, affiliation or non-affiliation with a multi-hospital system, standard metropolitan statistical area size, and region, are considered?

When other factors were held constant, the regression analysis found that there is no difference in the fractions of voluntary non-teaching and investor-owned hospitals charity and bad debt loads. Hospitals associated with the Council of Teaching Hospitals and public hospitals were found to have higher charity care/bad debt as a fraction of charges. In addition, hospitals in the south have higher uncompensated care loads than hospitals in the northeast, north-central or west census areas (Sloan, Valvona, and Mullner, 1984).

HCA Experience

HCA is committed to meeting the health care needs of its communities. Serving over 339 different cities nationwide, it provided 3.5 percent of gross revenue in uncompensated care through November 1983. The company recognizes that the need for uncompensated care depends on each community's unique circum-

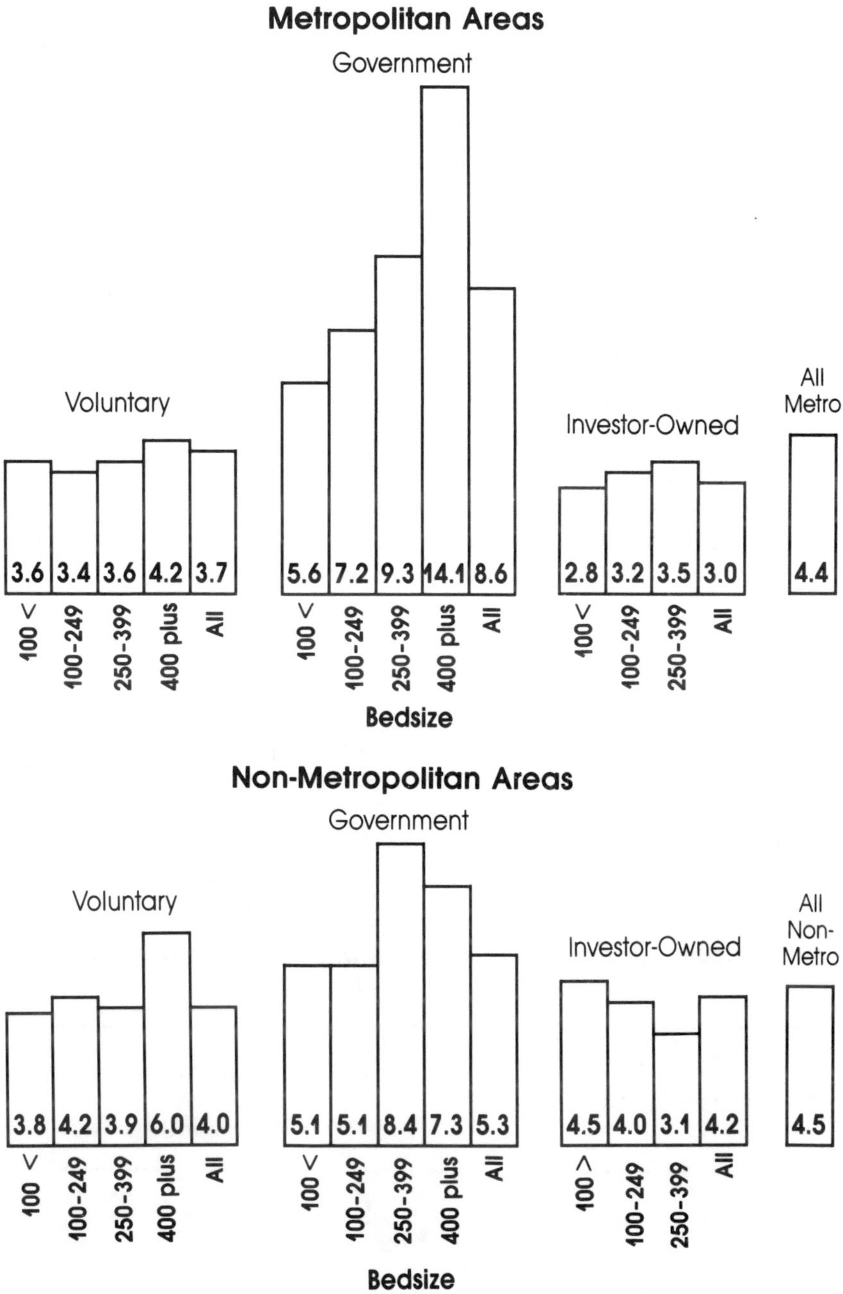

FIGURE 1. Uncompensated care as a Percent of Charges by location, ownership and bedsize, 1983

stances. For example, in communities where HCA is the sole provider, the percentage of uncompensated care is much higher than the company-wide percentage. As shown in Table 5, in Kentucky and Tennessee HCA's sole community hospitals provided an average of 4.8 percent of revenues in uncompensated care in 1983. When an HCA facility is one of several non-government hospitals, the amount of free care is more evenly distributed among providers. In these communities, HCA hospitals provided approximately 3.5 percent of total revenues. Last, in those communities with at least one tax supported public hospital, HCA's proportion of uncompensated care is appropriately less – 3.0 percent of total revenues.

While these figures do not compare HCA with its not-for-profit counterparts, they suggest that HCA's hospitals make a commitment to providing uncompensated care. The important point is that each hospital's commitment will vary, according to need and community resources, from full commitment in single-hospital towns to a sharing of uncompensated care loads in multiple-provider communities.

ACCESSIBILITY– FUNDING SOURCES

The investor-owned sector has made an impact on health services accessibility by creating pools that directly support the costs of indigent care. In January 1983, for example, Humana Corporation, the University of Louisville, the commonwealth of Kentucky,

TABLE 5
Uncompensated Care Provided At HCA Hospitals
January-November 1983

In Communities where*	As a Percentage of Gross Revenue
HCA is sole provider	4.8
Other non-government facilities exist	3.5
Public facilities exist	3.0

*Tennessee and Kentucky data.
Source: Hospital Corporation of America, Financial Data, 1983.

Jefferson County, and the city of Louisville reached a lease agreement that included the creation of a trust fund to provide reimbursement for indigent hospital care. Under the agreement, Humana Hospital University agreed to provide medically necessary care for all indigent and medically needy residents of Jefferson County. In return, the state, county, and city governments agreed to maintain their current level of indigent care funding and pool their monies into a trust fund specifically dedicated to charity care (Sloan, Valvona, and Mullner, 1984).

Upon the acquisition of public hospitals, HCA also has helped community governments to establish funding pools. Commonly, local governments will agree to continue their commitment to charity care by using hospital sales proceeds to establish and maintain an indigent care trust. These arrangements are frequently accompanied with an agreement by HCA to provide care for the poor.

While such funding pools are not necessarily limited to investor-owned involvement, they have been directly associated with the sale or lease of community hospitals. Funding pools represent one means by which local governments and investor-owned hospital companies can jointly establish a mechanism to finance and deliver care to the poor.

ACCESSIBILITY–OBLIGATION CONTRACTS

The investor-owned sector also has made an impact on health service accessibility by setting up and carrying out contract obligations to provide care for the disadvantaged. HCA's sales agreements, for example, often contain an explicit indigent care clause. These contractual arrangments vary from community to community. As an illustration, HCA agreed in one sales contract to provide care for all patients diagnosed as seriously ill or requiring emergency services without regard for the ability of such patients to pay. In return, the county agreed to reimburse the new HCA hospital for the costs of providing care to indigent patients to a contractual maximum amount per year. In another contract, HCA set a minimum indigent care obligation at two percent of its hospital's annual gross patient revenues, in addition to pledging never to refuse medically necessary emergency care to any person.

Contractual obligations are one measure of HCA's commitment to provide services to those unable to pay. Not only can such arrangements have a positive impact on access, but they also can eliminate some of the uncertainty associated with financing care for the poor.

A HOSPITAL'S APPROACH

At the heart of the question of the impact of investor-owned companies on access is what actually occurs at the community level. An illustration is provided by reviewing both the philosophy and actions of one 100-bed HCA facility located in Nashville, Tennessee (Fitzgerald, 1984).

With experience in both not-for-profit and investor-owned sectors, the administrator, John Fitzgerald, asserts that he sees little difference in behavior between ownership types regarding philosophy, management, and services offered. What little difference does exist, he believes, is limited to tax status, primarily in that investor-owned hospitals pay taxes while not-for-profits do not. Regarding the question of returns paid to stockholders, Mr. Fitzgerald responds that the dividends paid by investor-owned companies are no different than the returns not-for-profits pay to bond holders. He notes that the investor-owned companies do, in many respects, have the advantage of better access to capital. However, he believes that this difference is likely to decline in the future, especially as not-for-profit systems develop regionally and nationally.

Mr. Fitzgerald also states that while his hospital does not have an explicit policy on charity care, neither does it have maximum limits on the amount of uncompensated care offered. He adds that since the hospital has a full-service emergency room, it holds itself responsible for providing care in all life-threatening situations regardless of a person's ability to pay. Acting as a fiscally responsible business, the hospital will try to collect charges to the extent possible. Collection efforts, however, are handled on an individual basis according to a person's ability to pay.

Although the hospital does not open its doors indiscriminately to those who want free care, Mr. Fitzgerald believes that the hospital carries its fair share of uncompensated care. For example, according to hospital statistics reported to the state of Tennessee, his hospital provided 3.2 percent of uncompensated care in 1983 as a percentage of total patient revenue. This level is similar to the hospital's not-for-profit neighbors, including one religious hospital that provided 3.4 percent of total patient revenue in free care and another local not-for-profit hospital that provided 4.1 percent of total patient care revenue to those unable to pay. If taxes are included, the hospital's social responsibility amounted to 14.4 percent of total patient revenue in 1983.

Mr. Fitzgerald also notes that the county hospital, a tax-supported institution, provided 8.3 percent of total patient revenue in uncompensated care in 1983 – a level more than double that of the private hospitals studied. Although this figure is high compared with the private hospitals, he believes that the tax monies supporting public institutions should support social goals – most important, the goal of ensuring access for those unable to pay.

Regarding the issue of community-wide access, Mr. Fitzgerald comments that the hospital provides a number of outreach services common to its not-for-profit neighbors, such as health education, health promotion, and preventive services. These outreach programs, he believes, are an integral part of the hospital's mission to meet health care needs of the community residents.

The hospital's commitment to both community and indigent access directly contributes to its reputation as a quality institution. This is not to say that the actions exemplified by this HCA hospital are unique and should be applauded; however, it does point out that the hospital's actions are comparable to other private not-for-profits in the area.

SUMMARY

The evidence supports the conclusion that investor-owned hospitals are comparable to not-for-profit hospitals. In addition to similar behavior with respect to patient mix, service mix, and physician services, large investor-owned chains are able to bring capital, management expertise, and physician recruitment to hospital operations that positively impact the availability and accessibility of health services.

This does not mean that investor-owned hospitals are a solution to access problems. It is clear, however, that the evidence does not suggest that investor-owned hospitals are a cause of access problems. Patient dumping, market segmentation leading to disproportionate numbers of private patients in suburban hospitals, and long queues in hospital emergency rooms for indigent patients are common in many cities where there are no investor-owned hospitals (Knox, 1984). The problems associated with lack of accessibility to health care are not based on ownership.

Rather than looking at access from a good guy/bad guy perspective, we should focus on what is being done and what can be done to resolve access problems. At the hospital level, we need to acknowledge and encourage the balancing of economic and social objectives. This will be even more critical in light of our changing delivery system, in which significant pressures on hospitals increase demands for cost-effective care, enhance competition within the industry, and reduce ability to cross-subsidize uncompensated care by taxing those who are able to pay.

At a policy level, there are some fundamental questions to be addressed. The Federal Government has declared that health care is a right. This is a social objective that Americans accept and believe. Unfortunately, a practical approach for achieving that objective has not been developed. Medicare and Medicaid took a step in that direction; however, experience to date suggests that the problem is even bigger. Fundamentally, society must resolve many difficult issues before there is much hope of solving the access problem. A consensus must be developed on what we as a society are willing to pay for and how we want to pay for it.

While it is easy to shift the focus onto "society," many states and counties have taken initiatives within their own jurisdictions. Some of the innovative indigent care initiatives include (National Conference of State Legislators, 1984):

- **Risk-Sharing Pools** – Minnesota, Indiana, North Dakota, Wisconsin, Florida, Rhode Island have developed insurance risk-sharing pools to provide access to insurance for individuals who would otherwise have trouble obtaining coverage.
- **Health Insurance Premium Tax** –This approach would tax those who purchase health insurance. New Jersey has introduced legislation to finance catastrophic care for children by placing a surcharge on health insurance.
- **Prudent Buyer Plans** – Directing funds to targeted providers in return for providing indigent care is one way to establish a financing mechanism with built-in efficiency incentives. The Arizona and California Medicaid systems are two examples of the prudent buyer approach to uncompensated care.

We suspect that it will take more than local and state initiatives to address adequately the problems relating to access to health care. The real action lies in addressing questions such as:

- Will the emerging high-technology be available for medically indigent patients? (This includes access to organ transplants and artificial organs.)
- How explicitly will access be defined relative to amenity levels?
- Will limited groups of providers be tolerated? (The fears of a multi-tiered delivery system need to be addressed carefully.)
- Will the funding for non-paying patients be made explicit or left implicit as a cost shift?

Questions such as these are where the real challenges lie. Investor-owned hospitals have demonstrated the willingness to share a responsibility in meeting the social commitment to health care, but the true problems are currently bigger than a growing group of tax-paying hospitals.

APPENDIX A
Results of Regression Analysis on "Scope of Services" Measures B Coefficients and Standard Error of B

	Scope of Services			
Variables	Total Number of Services		Basic	
STATE				
Florida	.48	(.73)[1]	.02	(.07)
Tennessee	—		—	
Texas	1.02	(.50)*	.07	(.07)
California	4.56	(.54)**	.34	(.08)***
BED SIZE	.079	(.003)***	.004	(.0004)***
BED SIZE SQ	-5.2×10^{-5}	(.0000)***		
BED SHARE	1.01	(.59)	.08	(.10)
METRO	2.47	(.55)***	.008	(.07)
OWNERSHIP				
PUBLIC	—		—	
VOLUNTARY	.48	(.54)	−.16	(.08)*
IOC	1.62	(.75)*	−.10	(.13)
FIO	−2.38	(.57)***	.21	(.13)
VOLUNTARY METRO	−1.99	(.68)**	—	
FIO METRO	—		−.60	(.16)***
FIO BED SIZE	—		—	
IOC BED SIZE	−.017	(.004)***	−.0015	(.0006)*
VOL BED SHARE	—		—	
IOC BED SHARE	—		.40	(.19)*
Constant	11.2		2.67	
Multiple R^2	.72		.23	

*significant at 0.01 level
**significant at 0.05 level
***significant at 0.10 level
T values shown in parenthesis

REFERENCES

Annual Report to the Governor and State Legislature 1983–84. Tallahassee, FL, Hospital Cost Containment Board, March 1, 1984.

Berry, Ralph E. "On Grouping Hospitals for Economic Analysis," *Inquiry*, 10(4):5–13, December 1973.

Bryant, Dr. Rodney, Chief of Staff, Stones River Hospital. Personal Correspondence. March 19, 1984.

A Discursive Dictionary of Health Care. Subcommittee on Health and the Environment, U.S. House of Representatives. Washington, D.C., Government Printing Office, 1976.

Fitzgerald, John (Administrator, HCA). Personal Interview, September 18, 1984.

Gibson, Louis E. "Financing for Rural Hospitals," *Texas Hospitals*, 37(10):40–42, March 1982.

"HCFA Program Statistics," *Health Care Financing Review*, 4(2):165–170, December 1982.

The Hospital Cost Equation: It All Adds Up. Nashville, TN, Southeastern Hospital Conference, September 1983.

Hospital Management Industry Strategic Analysis. Sanford C. Bernstein and Co., Inc., New York, April 1983.

"Humana Leases Louisville University Hospital: To Provide Care for Needy," *FAH Review*, March/April 1983.

Knox, Richard A. "Some Local Hospitals 'Dump' the Uninsured," *The Boston Globe*, February 6, 1984, pp. 31, 33.

Lewin, Lawrence S., Derzon, Robert A., and Margulies, Rhea. "Investor-Owned and Non-profits Differ in Economic Performance," *Hospitals*, 55(13):52–58, July 1, 1981.

National Conference of State Legislators. *12 Questions: What Legislators Need to Know About Uncompensated Care*. Washington, D.C., National Conference of State Legislators, 1984.

Relman, Arnold S. "The New Medical-Industrial Complex." *The New England Journal of Medicine*, 303(17):963–970, October 23, 1980.

Shaw, Selm H. "Capital Access: The Compelling Issue of the '80s." *Equity Research Industry Comment*. New York, Shearson Lehman American Express, July 17, 1984.

Sloan, Frank A., Valvona, Joseph, and Mullner, Ross. "Identifying the Issues: A Statistical Profile." Draft paper presented at the Vanderbilt conference on *Uncompensated Care: Defining Rights and Assigning Responsibilities*. Nashville, TN, April 1984.

Sloan, Frank A. and Vraciu, Robert A. "Investor-Owned and Not-For-Profit Hospitals: Addressing Some Issues." *Health Affairs*, 2(1):25–37, Spring 1983.

STEPHEN M. SHORTELL, PH.D.
A. C. Buehler Distinguished Professor of Hospital and Health Management and Professor of Organization Behavior, J. L. Kellogg Graduate School of Management and Center for Health Services and Policy Research, Northwestern University, Evanston, Illinois

Implications of Hospital Ownership on Access to Care

As concern over the soaring costs of health care increases, many believe we have abandoned our commitment to improve the nation's access to health services evidenced in the social programs of the 1960s and 1970s. I maintain that this was a half-hearted commitment at best, and that as a nation we have never faced up to the issue of making available a basic set of health services to all Americans, however comprehensive or restrictive those services may be. Some salient points include the following (McNerney, 1983):

1. Medicaid eligibility requirements and benefits still vary significantly by state with associated problems for targeted populations.
2. The difference betweeen protection and non-protection is thin and sometimes arbitrarily drawn; for example, under Medicaid a child in a one-parent household may be eligible while one in a two-parent household is not.
3. Many low income individuals without Medicaid coverage still have no health insurance, while others have weak protection highly dependent on employment and often in industries with low fringe benefits.
4. Medicaid enrollment fell between 1975 and 1979, and further cutbacks were made in 1983.

5. The proportion of the total health bill paid for by Medicare has been steadily falling since 1965.
6. Many public and private hospitals in the inner cities no longer exist. Numerous public hospitals have been closed in the past few years, and some private hospitals have moved to the suburbs.
7. Community health centers with the potential to address the special needs of the poor and tailored to local needs have suffered recent budget cuts despite impressive impacts on some dimensions of health status. Thus, low-income groups have been deprived of this alternative service.
8. Research indicates that early gains of the poor and physician visits adjusted for chronic illness by age group are leveling off and that physician visits per 100 disability days for the poor showed no gains during the 1970s (Aday and Andersen, 1981).
9. Non-whites with Medicare coverage are 30 percent less likely to be admitted to nursing homes than whites for covered services (Public Health Service, 1980).
10. The insured receive 54 percent more ambulatory care than the uninsured and 90 percent more hospital care than the uninsured (Davis, 1982).
11. The number of uninsured poor is increasing while hospital free care is decreasing. For example, between 1980 and 1982, 13.5 percent of the population was living at least 150 percent below the poverty line, and 21 percent were inadequately insured. However, during the same period, public and private hospitals' proportion of free care increased only 3.8 percent (Hospital Week, 1984).

These data suggest that the access issue is much larger than merely whether differences in hospital ownership may be systematically associated with differences in access to care. We are looking at a relatively small piece of the puzzle. What makes the topic particularly significant, however, is that the growing rationing of health care is beginning to affect the large middle-class segment of the population and not just the poor. Thus, an examination of how organizational forms may interact with changes in third-party coverage and hospital payment is particularly opportune.

In this paper, I attempt four things. First, I will try to clarify what is meant by *access*. Second, I will discuss those factors that have been shown to be associated with differences in access to care.

Third, I will summarize what we know about the relationship between hospital ownership forms and access to care. And finally, I will suggest some questions, issues, and approaches for further study.

WHAT IS ACCESS TO CARE?

There are many definitions of access in the literature, ranging from the availability of services and the ease of entry into the system to the measurement of the actual utilization of services relative to need (Aday and Andersen, 1974). For purposes of this discussion, we will define access simply as the ability to obtain health care services when needed. This may, of course, be restricted by the lack of available providers, facilities, or related services; by lack of financial coverage; or by psychological, social, geographic, and organizational barriers. These dimensions raise the issue of what constitutes "adequate" access to care, an issue that is further confounded by varying definitions of medical need – for example, as perceived by the individual or as determined by professional medical judgment.

The issue of access is of interest in relation to the quality of services that individuals receive to restore or enhance their health. This adds a new area of growing public concern: namely, whether we are moving closer to a two-tier system of care – one for the well-off and well-insured and the other for the poor and uninsured. I think the issue can be sharpened by considering quality and scope of services on the one hand and access on the other, as shown in Figure 1.

In Figure 1, the "ideal" state is represented by a high degree of both access and quality. Such a situation is enjoyed by those with good insurance coverage, living in areas with a ready supply of well-trained providers. The "two-class" state is represented by a relatively high degree of access but with relatively low quality and limited supply of services. This might include residents in inner city areas who have access only to the chronically under-staffed public hospital. The "rationing" state is represented by poor access to high-quality services. This is different from the two-class state in that individuals potentially receive the same quality and scope of services as everyone else, but the system limits or rations the number of individuals who can receive such care. Rationing may occur through the use of co-insurance and deductibles as well as through the behavior of providers and institutions. For example, well-off suburban hospitals, through pricing and admission policies, may discourage certain groups of patients from receiving care. The fourth state, "neglect," is characterized by both low access and low quality and scope of

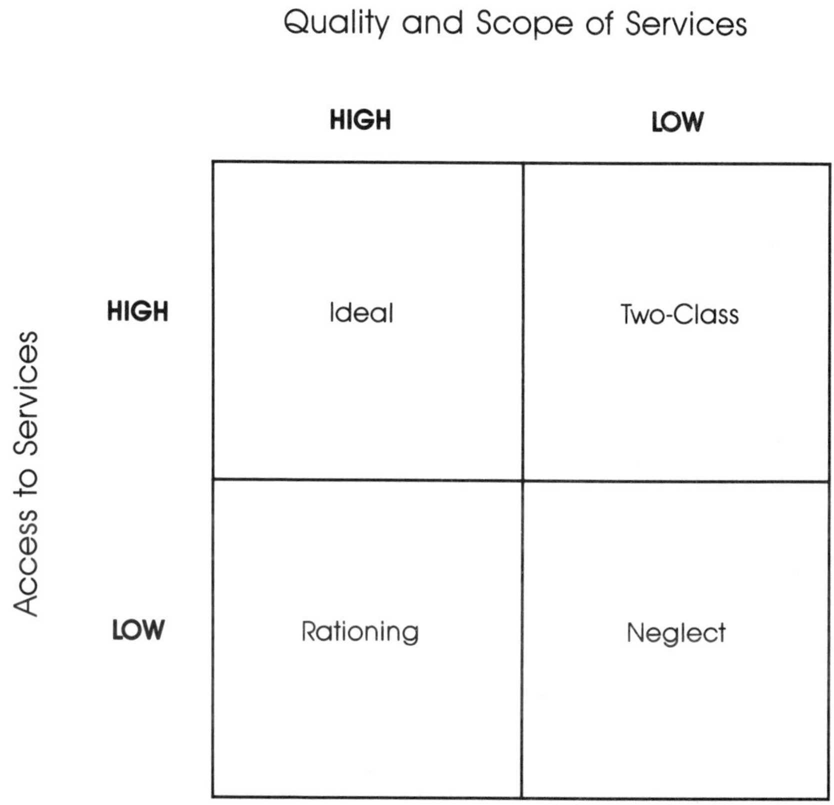

FIGURE 1. A typology of access to care.

Source: Shortell, S. M., Wickizer, T. M. and Wheeler, J. R. C., Jr., *Hospital-Physician Joint Ventures: Results and Lessons from a National Demonstration in Primary Care.* Ann Arbor, Michigan: Health Administration Press, 1984.

services provided. Examples include residents living in some rural and selected inner city areas of the country.

From a policy perspective, one can examine the distribution of certain groups (e.g., the poor, near poor, middle class, rural versus urban, insured versus non-insured) across the four cells shown. I suggest that we should focus our concern on the neglect and rationing cells rather than on the two-class cell. Individuals in the two-class cell at least have access to some set of health services, but those in the rationing state have a high probability of receiving no care at all, even though the facilities, services, and providers in their area may be of high quality. Obviously, this is an oversimplification because the situations greatly depend on the specific needs of the people involved. But the figure enables us to consider access in a broader perspective. What strategies, policies, and management practices (such as pricing, transfer policies, and location decisions) of different types of hospitals might be related to the rationing of services, creation of multiple tiers or levels of service, and outright neglect? To consider this issue in perspective, we must briefly review those factors that have been found to be associated with differences in access.

FACTORS ASSOCIATED WITH DIFFERENCES IN ACCESS

Demographic, psychosocial, economic, and organizational factors have all been found to be associated to some extent with differences in access (Shortell, 1984). Demographic factors include age, sex, race, marital status, family size, social class, education, and occupation. Psychosocial factors include health beliefs, values, norms, attitudes, and culture. Economic dimensions include income, insurance coverage, price and provider and facility/population ratios. Among the organizational factors that have been considered to date are the use of health maintenance organizations (HMOs) and prepaid group practices, referral patterns, and the presence of a regular source of care. Much of the existing research suggests that the economic factors (particularly insurance coverage) are most consistently and strongly related to differences in utilization and to the ability of prepaid group practices or HMOs to reduce the volume of hospital utilization. In the latter regard, one might raise the interesting question of whether this represents less access to needed secondary and tertiary care. Conspicuously missing from the above findings is any mention of ownership or the organization of hospitals. In what way may these factors influence access to care, and are there any studies outside the main access/utilization literature to guide us?

THE ROLE AND EVIDENCE REGARDING HOSPITAL ORGANIZATION AND OWNERSHIP

How Might Systems Facilitate Access?

A major development in health care during the past ten years has been the growth in the number of hospitals belonging to multi-unit systems, both investor-owned and voluntary not-for-profit (Ermann and Gabel, 1984). There are three main ways in which systems might improve access to care: (1) by making use of their greater financial resources and access to capital markets (in the latter regard, particularly the investor-owned); (2) by making use of their management and personnel; and (3) by achieving economies of scale. Systems can use their greater financial resources and access to capital to start new services needed by the community, maintain existing needed services that are losing money, subsidize inner city or rural hospitals serving the poor, recruit physicians and other health professionals, and provide improvements in equipment and technology. Systems can use their greater personnel resources to improve the efficiency and effectiveness with which services are provided to the community (this could result in reduced waiting time for appointments, reduced office waiting time, and more efficient delivery of services) and to upgrade the technical skills of physicians, nurses, and other health professionals through conducting clinical educational programs and sharing clinical resources. Systems could use economies of scale in purchasing and related areas to make it easier for hospitals to obtain certain supplies and other resources for service development and enhancement in their local areas.

How Might Systems Hinder Access?

Under cost-containment pressures, all hospitals must reexamine the services they offer their patients. Each service needs to be viewed in terms of its profitability, current market share, and potential growth in market share, in addition to its technical quality and the degree to which it meets defined community needs. However, unlike individual free-standing hospitals, the decisions of systems may have more pervasive influences. The key factor involves the way in which these decisions are made and their outcomes in regard to certain macro and micro issues. Specifically, highly centralized systems may make decisions at the corporate office level that do not take into account local need or are not sensitive to local wishes and, thus, may impair access to care. These may involve macro decisions, such as the acquisition or divestiture of a hospital, or micro decisions, such as the addition or deletion of specific services. A major concern with the acquisition decision is whether the system will continue to maintain existing services desired by the community and to serve existing patient groups desiring those services. A major concern with the divestiture decision is whether the system has discerned that alternative providers are available in the community to meet adequately patient needs before deciding to pull out. Similar considerations arise in regard to specific service lines, such as the deletion of unprofitable services that may still be needed by the community. In brief, systems can use their strategies, policies, and practices to promote or impair access by making more or fewer providers, facilities, and services available to defined population groups and by making it more or less difficult to make contact with the available facilities, providers, and services. What is the evidence to date?

The Evidence Regarding the Effect of Hospital Organization and Ownership

There is relatively little evidence regarding the influence of system organization or invester-owned versus voluntary ownership on access to care. Most of what we know comes from studies by Lewin and Associates (1976), Pattison and Katz (1983), and Sloan and Vraciu (1983), and the research synthesis of Ermann and Gabel (1984). These studies suggest no significant national differences between investor-owned system hospitals and voluntary free-standing hospitals in regard to the percentage of Medicare and Medicaid patients served, the percentage of charity or indigent care delivered, or the scope of services offered to the community. However, a recent study suggests that in selected states (for example, Tennessee and Texas) investor-owned hospitals provide less uncompensated care than voluntary not-for-profit hospitals (I.O.M., 1985). Data developed by the National Health Law Program Clearing House (Dallek, 1983) also suggest that investor-owned hospitals provide less uncompensated care, but these data are not adjusted for hospital size, region of the country, or related variables.

In regard to serving the Medicaid, the poor, as well as the general provision of charity care, the major difference is not between investor-owned and voluntary hospitals but rather between these and public hospitals (Homer, Bradham and Rushefsky, 1984; Schlesinger and Dorwat, 1984). For example, a recent California study indicated that the estimated cost of hospital bad debt and charity care per patient day during 1980 and 1981 was $115 for county hospitals, $16 for secular non-profit hospitals, $12 for investor-owned hospitals, $12 for district hospitals, and $11 for religiously affiliated non-profit hospitals (California Association of Public Hospitals, 1984). It is the public hospitals in this country that bear the disproportionate burden of providing uncompensated care.

It is important to note that none of the existing work explicitly compares investor-owned system hospitals with voluntary *system* hospitals to determine whether there really is an ownership effect separate from a system effect. Nor have there been comparisons of *both* voluntary system and investor-owned system hospitals with free-standing hospitals to assess the *system* affect on access independent of ownership.

Recent case studies suggest that investor-owned systems do make arrangements to continue to provide equivalent amounts of uncompensated care as existed before the takeover (Townsend, 1983). In contrast, preliminary data from a study of a hospital acquisition in Florida suggest that the percentage of uncompensated care provided declines after acquisition by an investor-owned company (Brown and Klosterman, 1984). However, it is not known whether this is due to fewer poor patients being served or to more aggressive payment and collection policies to reduce bad debts. Clearly, the issue requires further study with emphasis on determining the conditions and circumstances under which more-or-less uncompensated care may be provided after acquisition. The issue will become even more important as the voluntary non-profit systems also increase their acquisition activities.

The existing works focus only on the types of patients served and, to some extent, services offered. They do not address such issues as waiting time to get an appointment, the waiting time in the outpatient department or ambulatory care center, travel distance, or the percentage of patients transferred to other hospitals or sources of care (Himmelstein, et al., 1984). These represent areas for future study and are discussed in the following section.

ISSUES AND QUESTIONS: A RESEARCH AGENDA FOR THE FUTURE

Recognizing that the access issue is primarily a national health financing policy issue, we have considered what it is that the individual hospitals and systems might do to provide or impair access. To some extent, we already addressed these concerns, but our focus here lies more in the future than in the past. Some possibilities include the following:

1. Expand services into areas of the country currently demanding or needing such services, such as the federally designated Health Manpower Shortage Areas.
2. Maintain currently unprofitable but needed service lines where no alternative providers exist.
3. Develop service lines to meet newly identified market needs, particularly in regard to disease prevention/health promotion

and out-of-hospital services representing less costly alternatives for care.

4. Set aside a predetermined percentage of profits for the direct provision of charity care or for a fund supporting such care by the public hospital or other providers in the community (a version of the latter is currently being tried in Florida).
5. Develop management systems and practices to provide more cost-effective care resulting in less costly care, a lower increase in premiums, and greater financial accessibility.

Given limited resources, all hospitals will be considering these possibilities within the context of trade-offs that might be made. It is a popular notion that the pressures on hospitals to contain costs will result in diminished access to care and quality of care. But we should at least entertain the idea that in some cases or for certain conditions access and quality might improve. For example, as hospitals develop more outpatient services and reduce their inpatient capacities to compete more effectively under prospective payment, they bring care closer to patients, making such services not only less costly than if provided in an inpatient setting but also more convenient. In other cases, restricting access to care by providing certain technologies and services in a limited number of sites may actually improve the quality of care by providing a sufficient volume of patients to promote technical competence (Luft, Bunker and Enthoven, 1979; Shortell and LoGerfo, 1981). Thus, we need to consider access not in a vacuum but in relation to cost, quality, and other considerations. A suggested framework is shown in Figure 2.

This figure shows a number of possible interrelationships among patient characteristics, provider/system characteristics, access, utilization, continuity, cost, quality of care, and patient satisfaction. For our purposes, it is sufficient to note that the framework permits assessment of possible trade-offs that may exist among access, cost, quality, and related dimensions of health service and, in turn, how these may be associated with differences in hospital organization and ownership as well as related variables. Given this framework, the following kinds of studies might be considered:

1. Community household-based surveys of utilization and access to care in areas with a variety of investor-owned and voluntary system hospitals, free-standing hospitals, and public hospitals would enable researchers to examine differences in utilization, waiting times, travel distance and times, and satisfaction with care among people using different kinds of

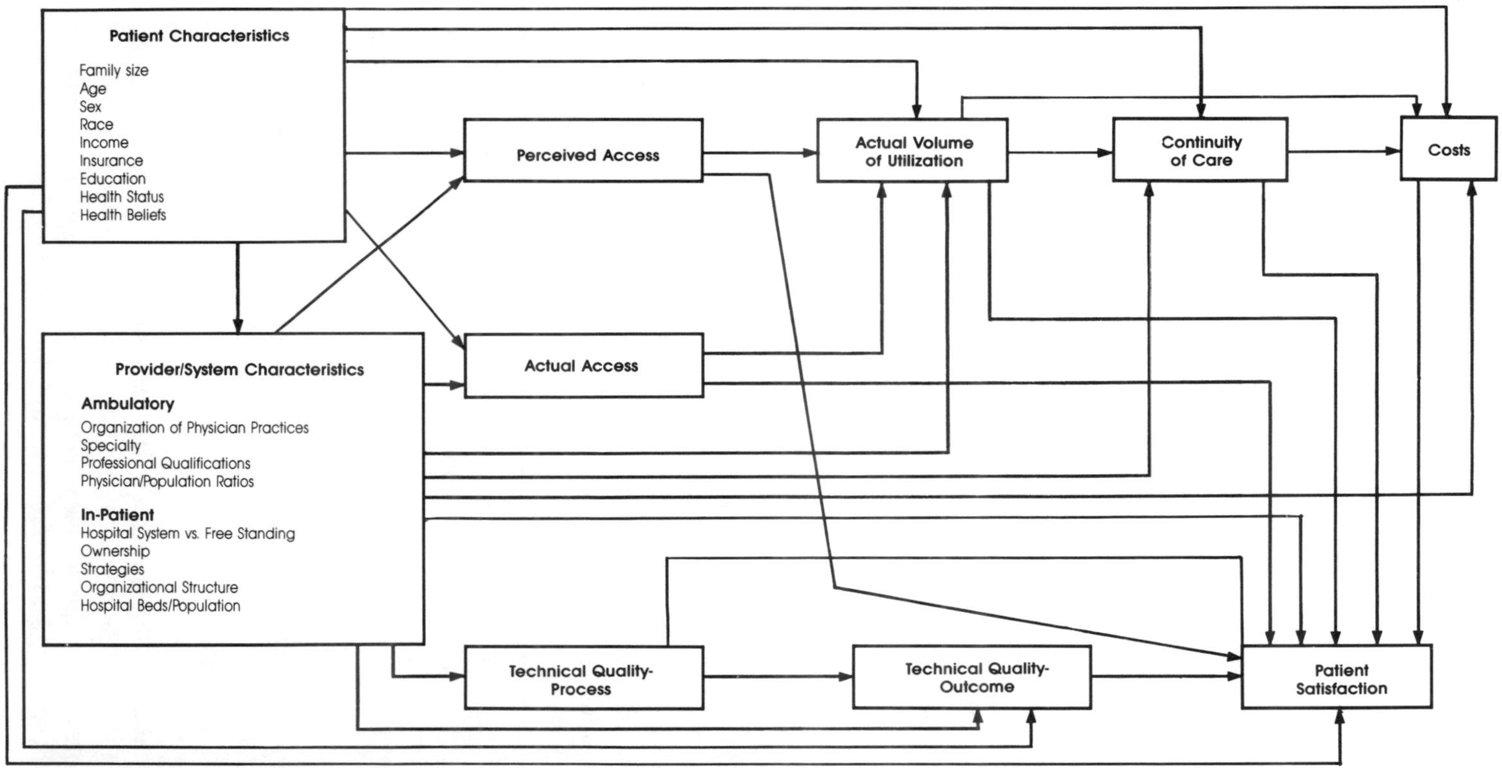

Source: Expanded from Shortell, S. M., Richardson, W. C., LoGerfo, J. P., et. al.: The Relationships Among Dimensions of Health Services in Two Provider Systems: A Casual Model Approach. *Journal of Health and Social Behavior*, 18:139–159, June 1977.

FIGURE 2. Causal model of dimensions of health services provision.

hospitals. This would require that the respondent information be directly linked to the hospital used, including not only in-patient care but also out-of-hospital services that are associated with a specific hospital.

2. Community household-based surveys examining the above issues could also be carried out in communities dominated by investor-owned system hospitals versus voluntary system hospitals versus free-standing hospitals.
3. Studies could be conducted examining the pre- and post-prospective payment shifts in out-of-hospital services offered by investor-owned system hospitals, voluntary system hospitals, free-standing hospitals, and public hospitals. Such studies should be based on defined community market areas so that the effects could be assessed of a change in policy or strategy or service mix of one hospital on the strategies, policies and service mix of other hospitals in the community or market area.
4. Longitudinal studies should be conducted of system acquisitions of other hospitals over time. What services are added, deleted, or maintained and for what population groups? How might this differ depending on the number and type of other hospitals in the area? Similar studies should be done in regard to the divestiture of hospitals. Briefly, what happens to these hospitals and their communities after they are "dropped" by a given hospital system?
5. Local studies of patient transfers among hospitals should be conducted (Himmelstein, et al., 1984). Methodologies would have to be worked out to assess accurately what constitutes a transfer of a patient from one hospital to another. Distinctions would need to be made between voluntary and involuntary transfers, taking into account presenting conditions, geographic distance between the patient's residence and the original contacting hospital versus the eventual providing hospital, and so on.
6. Studies should isolate the effect of competition on the number and type of services rendered to various population groups. One might expect the greatest changes in service mix and volume under conditions of high competition among hospitals in specific areas. In other words, it is not just cost-containment that is driving changes in the provision of services but rather, the interaction of cost-containment policies with other factors such as the degree of competition among hospitals, among physicians, and between hospitals and physicians.

7. The influence of hospital strategies and policies on the provision of services to various groups should be explored. To what degree are different kinds of hospitals pursuing market penetration versus market development strategies; product refinement versus new product development strategies; and strategies of acquisition versus growth from within? Such studies would provide some real insight into the operation of both investor-owned and voluntary system hospitals. The ownership distinction alone is too simplistic and won't lead us very far. We need to look at the underlying strategies and policies that systems pursue. It is possible, for example, that there may be as much within-ownership variance as between-ownership variance in terms of access issues.

SUMMARY

We have reviewed what is meant by access to care, discussed factors associated with differences in access, considered the role and evidence pertaining to the influence of hospital organization and ownership on access to care, and identified several issues and areas for further study. Three points were highlighted. First, access is primarily a national health financing policy issue, not a hospital ownership issue. Second, access must be considered within a broad framework that simultaneously takes into account cost, quality, and related considerations. Third, the underlying strategies, incentives, and policies of all hospitals must be examined. It cannot be assumed that these factors can be understood adequately by simplistic ownership distinctions as if ownership alone was a valid proxy variable for hospital behavior.

REFERENCES

Aday, L. A. and Andersen, R. "A Framework for the Study of Access to Medical Care." *Health Services Research*, 9(3):208–220, Fall 1974.

Aday, L. A., and Andersen, R. M. "Equity of Access to Medical Care: A Conceptual and Empirical Overview." *Medical Care*, 19(12):4–27 (Supplement), December 1981.

Brown, K. J. and Klosterman, R. E. "Hospital Acquisitions and Their Effects: An Analysis of Florida Data, 1979-1982," Draft Paper Prepared for the Insitute of Medicine's Committee on the For-Profit Role in Health Care, National Academy of Sciences, August 15, 1984.

California Association of Public Hospitals "Health Care in the 80s – Can the Safety Net Survive?" White Paper on the Unique Contributions and Needs of California's Public Hospitals, 1984.

Dallek, G. "For-Profit Hospitals and the Poor." *Clearing House Review*, 17(8):860–867, December 1983.

Davis, K. "Access to Amulatory Care: Public Policy Implications." Paper presented at the Brandeis University Conference on the Cost of Ambulatory Care, Key Biscayne, Florida, June 6–9, 1982.

Ermann, D. and Gabel, J. "Multihospital Systems: Issues and Empirical Findings." *Health Affairs*, 3(1):50–64, Spring 1984.

Himmelstein, D. V., et al. "Patient Transfers: Medical Practice as Social Triage." *American Journal of Public Health*, 74(5):494--497, May 1984.

Homer, C. G., Bradham, D. D., and Rushefsky, M. "Investor-Owned and Not-For-Profit Hospitals: Beyond the Cost and Revenue Debate." *Health Affairs*, 3(4):133–136, Winter 1984.

Hospital Week. 20(26), June 29, 1984.

Institute of Medicine, National Academy of Science, *Report on the For-Profit Role in Health Care*, forthcoming.

Lewin and Associates. *A Study of Investor-Owned Hospitals*, unpublished Report to Health Services Foundation, 1976.

Luft, H., Bunker, J. P., and Enthoven, A. C. "Should Operations be Regionalized? The Empirical Relation Between Surgical Volume and Mortality." *The New England Journal of Medicine*, 301(25):1364–1369, December 20, 1979.

McNerney, W. J. "A Two-Tier System of Health Care." Duke University Forum, Durham, North Carolina, March 14, 1983.

Pattison, R. and Katz, H. "Investor-Owned and Not-For-Profit Hospitals: A Comparison Based on California Data." *The New England Journal of Medicine*, 309(6):347–353, August 11, 1983.

Public Health Service, Office of Health Resources Opportunity. "Health of the Disadvantaged." *Chartbook-2*, 1980, pp. 68-69.

Schlesinger, M. and Dorwart, R. "Ownership and Mental Health Services: A Reappraisal of the Shift Toward Privately Owned Facilities." *The New England Journal of Medicine*, 311(15):959--965, October 1984.

Shortell, S. M. "Factors Associated with the Use of Health Services." Williams, S. J., and Torrens, P. R. (Eds.), *Introduction to Health Services*, Second Edition. New York: John Wiley & Sons, 1984.

Shortell, S. M. and LoGerfo, J. P. "Hospital Medical Staff Organization and Quality of Care: Results For Myocardial Infarction and Appendectomy." *Medical Care*, 19(10):1041–1056, October 1981.

Sloan, F. and Vraciu, R. "Investor-Owned and Not-For-Profit Hospitals: Addressing Some Issues." *Health Affairs*, 2(1):25–37, Spring 1983.

Townsend, J. "When Investor-Owned Corporations Buy Hospitals: Some Issues and Concerns." Gray, B. (Ed.), *The New Health Care For-Profit*. Washington, D.C.: Institute of Medicine, National Academy of Sciences, 1983.

Basil J. F. Mott Ph.D.
Dean,
School of Health Studies,
University of New Hampshire

Whither the Soul of Health Care?

We are on an uncertain historical voyage of unprecedented sweeping change in health care. We are experiencing basic changes in how health care is organized, delivered, financed, and to whom services are provided. I think most of us would agree that no one knows how it all will end. Although I hold a particular point of view, I welcome examination of my premises and values.

I believe many – perhaps most – of the changes taking place are for the good. For example, things are being done to improve the quality of health care by decreasing unnecessary utilization and hospitalization. The drain on the nation's resources is being reduced by providing health care in more cost-effective ways. Moreover, wellness is being promoted by fostering values that call for Americans to take greater responsibility for their own health.

But in our anxiousness to adapt to the environment to ensure the survival of our institutions, we risk transformations that could severely damage the American health care system, which I believe is the best in the world. We risk losing some of the basic values that have been at the core of health care, that have given it special meaning, purpose, and direction. I refer to the moral responsibility to serve people and to the charitable values that come from our religious heritage, which are best reflected in the belief that health care is a right. We may lose sight of our responsibility to care for the poor, the sick, and the disabled. It is more than just a matter of serving people. (Perhaps a hospital shouldn't even exist that is moved only by the drive for survival and organizational maintenance.) It is a matter of doing good. It *is* a matter of being our brother's keeper.

With the weakening of these values, there is risk to hospitals as institutions in which people place special trust because they believe they exist for them, and thus to hospitals as social institutions. There is also risk to hospitals as community institutions that reflect community values. I refer to "noblesse oblige," the moral obligation felt by community leaders to serve their communities and to help others less fortunate than they.

I must acknowledge that we and our hospitals have often fallen short in living up to our traditional values. But if we make it more difficult to attain our ideals, or lose faith in them, I believe there will be a grave risk to the heart and soul of health care.

I have divided the sources of risk into three areas and shall discuss each briefly: business management, commercialization of health care, and multi-hospital systems.

BUSINESS MANAGEMENT

The introduction of methods of business management is of great benefit to our hospitals and other health institutions (e.g., strategic planning, productivity measures, marketing, sophisticated cost-analysis systems, and corporate reorganization). In many respects, these managerial techniques are essential to non-profit groups as well as to investor-owned institutions. There are, however, serious risks in the adoption of business methods, about which we may not be sufficiently aware. There is a certain seductiveness about a business orientation and the corporate world. Hospital administrators, trustees, and physicians can get caught up in the excitement of launching new ventures, developing health care empires, and in being part of the world of organization, finance, and legal restructuring, and thereby lose sight of what health care is all about. Means may become ends because of their attractiveness. To caricature the scene, some of us may take an "ego-trip" in the world of entrepreneurship and high finance, drawn by the glamour of the corporate office and the corporate jet whisking us around as we build new corporations and service networks.

Even the language of hospital administrators and trustees suggests that we may be adopting beliefs that are antithetical to the values of service and caring. I speak of such abstract and tough talk as strategy, tactics, market penetration, and product realignment – jargon that depicts a world of winners and losers, a macho world that is like war. It isn't a language that evokes the values of serving and caring for human beings. Let me quote Karl Weick of Cornell, (Peters and Waterman, 1984), a well known contemporary writer on management theory who is concerned about the overuse of the military analogy in the business world: "Organizations have staff, line, and chain of command. They develop strategy and tactics. Organizations attack competitors, recruit MBAs. . . . They solve problems by discharging people (honorably or otherwise), tightening controls, introducing discipline, sending for reinforcements, or clarifying responsibilities – since that's what you do when an army sags," (p. 101). I do not intend to poke fun, except to make a point. We may gradually be slipping into a view of the health world that undermines the values of caring for people who are sick and dying.

Surprisingly, we may be adopting a view of management that is losing favor in the business world. In their book *In Search of Excellence*, Peters and Waterman (1984) report that leading thinkers are departing radically from past views and that this is reflected in a shift away from the military analogy, which Karl Weick argues limits our ability to think sensibly about management problems and thus to solve them effectively.

Robert Sigmond, in a speech entitled "Social Implications of New Business Strategies for Health Care Corporations", (1984), said that businesses may have as much to learn from well-run hospitals as hospitals have to learn from businesses. He points out that good hospitals possess at least six of the eight characteristics that Peters and Waterman cite as attributes of excellent corporations, including a strong value system. Therefore, hospitals don't need to be tight, disciplined organizations; they are infused with values that guide the performance of their members.

Sigmond goes further and points out that the meaning of what is "business-like" is also in question. What is meant by a "business orientation" in health care? Profits? A good accounting system? An efficient operation? We are seldom clear when we call for businesslike practices.

The world of business poses another risk to hospitals. It simply may be too appealing to some hospital administrators. They may see its forms and methods as a way to increase their status and power, to make them more professional, and to give them greater control over their medical staffs. Those of us who have been, or are, hospital administrators know that heading an organization with a medical staff and a lay board of trustees is one of the most difficult managerial positions in our society. Hospital administrators must maintain the support of a medical staff over whom they have little formal authority (indeed, whose members view administrators as a threat to their autonomy), and they must account to people who have little understanding of physicians and of the workings of hospitals. Some administrators seek the transformation of their boards along corporate lines by changing trustees into paid directors and by installing inside directors from management. As a trustee, I am very uncomfortable with these ideas, which I believe could mean the end of the dedicated volunteer serving his or her community. As paid directors, how could we represent our community or testify on behalf of our hospital before a legislative body with any more credibility than our Chief Executive Officer? Moreover, can trustees be paid enough to make it meaningful?

There is a risk to the health field at an even more fundamental level. In adopting the ways of business management, we may confuse management with institutional leadership. Management is essentially concerned with efficiency, about getting things done cost-effectively. Leadership, on the other hand, is concerned with the promotion and protection of values. To quote Philip Selznick, (1950), one of the finest writers on the subject of management and leadership, and to whom Peters and Waterman turn as a seminal writer, "Leadership . . . fails when it concentrates on sheer survival: institutional survival properly understood is a matter of maintaining values and distinctive identity." (p. 63)

COMMERCIALIZATION OF HEALTH CARE

I shall now turn to the commercialization of health care. As Eli Ginzberg made clear in a May 1984 article in *The New England Journal of Medicine*, health care is being drawn increasingly and fully into the economy. In becoming money based, however, which is probably unavoidable, there is a danger that it will become money driven. There is a risk that health care will become a fully commercialized product, marketed out of the need for profit to satisfy investors, which is, of course, appropriate and necessary in a business. Voluntary, as well as investor-owned, hospitals are threatened by this. Through unrestrained entrepreneurship, hospitals may come to view health care as a commodity to be marketed, much as other goods and services.

To the extent that health care is treated as a marketed commodity, we face the issue of how to protect its inherent values when they conflict with the values of commerce. In discussing some of the questions involved, I shall draw upon some of the ideas in Robert Veatch's article in the book, *New Health Care for Profit.*

First, we must ask ourselves how we are going to resist excluding unprofitable customers (e.g., a poor or middle class person who needs but cannot afford open heart surgery). Businesses exclude them, and they should; they do not have a moral obligation to serve unprofitable customers.

How are we going to continue supplying unprofitable services needed by the community? In the past, we have believed that a hospital had an obligation to try to meet the community's needs. It is not, however, in the interests of a business to supply unprofitable services, unless it is compelled to do so (e.g., by a regulatory body).

Third, how can we avoid enticing needless consumption? Sears Roebuck doesn't care if I buy six tires when I only need four; in fact, it would gladly sell me a dozen. That does not make Sears the slightest bit unethical. It doesn't have an obligation to be concerned about the quantity of products or services I buy. It has an obligation only to present for sale quality products in an ethical way.

Finally, how can we protect physicians from pressures to serve corporate objectives when they conflict with professional values, namely, the physician's obligation to place the patient's interests above all others.

In confronting these questions, it appears that investor-owned hospitals have the most difficult task. They face the problem of balancing the needs of their stockholders against the social purposes that we expect hospitals to serve.

There also is some doubt that physicians will be able to resist successfully the full commercialization of health care, and thus whether the entrepreneurial side of medicine will overwhelm its character as a calling. Are we heading toward the day when physicians will feel less and less of an obligation to care for people unless doing so involves a monetary transaction that is favorable to them? The physician participating in profitable joint ventures, the physician setting up his or her own business, the physician owning the service to which he or she refers patients–all raise ethical questions as important as any medicine has ever faced.

Most of us probably would agree that we won't know the answers to these questions for a decade or more, although by then the die may be cast. To try to answer them now would be as dogmatic as to deny their importance. For example, we do not know how well the Joint Committee on Accreditation of Hospitals (JCAH) and the courts will protect access to care and the quality of care from economic pressures. And we do not know how aging of the investor-owned hospitals, or a change in the balance of investor-owned vs. voluntary hospitals–if it occurs–will affect the performance of for-profit and not-for-profit hospitals.

MULTI-HOSPITAL SYSTEMS

Notwithstanding the many benefits of multi-hospital systems (e.g., their access to capital and to managerial talent), they may undermine the community roots of hospitals. Inevitably, when hospitals are drawn into a national or regional system, there is a risk to community values (e.g., to the values implicit in community governance by a voluntary board of trustees drawn from the community). Traditionally, our hospitals have been community oriented institutions. Much of their strength derives from their community roots. Multi-hospital systems are likely to weaken this attachment when corporate goals conflict with community needs and values. This issue raises a number of questions. Can mutually acceptable compromises between corporate and community interests be reached? Will investor-owned chains pull out of communities that are unprofitable? If so, will they sell their institutions to investors having little concern about community interests?

It is generally not in the interest of a business to care to whom it sells, except when its reputation may be adversely affected. We have many examples of large American corporations, such as steel and automobile companies, abandoning American communities for more profitable locations, which is a reasonable course from their point of view. Can we expect different social performance from profit-making health institutions? Will the voluntary multi-hospital systems behave differently when they need to close or get rid of a hospital that is losing money?

We must also consider the effect on the governance of hospitals and, thereby, voluntarism, which is people serving community institutions through a belief in social responsibility. If we lose the values of voluntarism, will our view of hospitals change?

Moreover, will hospitals that belong to multi-hospital systems be good community neighbors? Will their corporate headquarters allow them to be responsible community citizens (e.g., by participating in health coalitions and planning with other health agencies)? Sigmond (1984) believes the investor-owned hospitals face a dilemma in this regard that they must resolve in the interests of their stockholders.

CONCLUSIONS

In raising these issues, I want to make it clear that I am not suggesting we can go backwards. In my own hospital, I am involved in corporate restructuring, including efforts that are leading to profit-making enterprises. I believe, however, that we have some choice over how things will work out and that how we exercise our options may make the difference, at least enough difference to give us confidence we have shaped the best possible future. I do not believe we are faced with an absolute determinism. I find troubling the uncritical acceptance of projections and trends, as if they usually were more than educated guesses. In fact, they can become self-fulfilling prophecies, if we accept them as gospel. Who would have predicted the passage of prospective pricing within months of the Tax Equity Fiscal Responsibility Act?

Our hospitals are special and unique institutions that have been shaped by the moral and religious values of service to people, which is the underlying basis of the public's trust in them. What our hospitals become in the future will depend largely on the values we hold and the leadership we provide our institutions. At a recent national meeting, a distinguished administrator said, "The values of a health organization and of its executives are the basis of leadership." (Connors, 1984). At the same meeting another health leader challenged the participants with the observation, "Surprisingly we (in the health field) are embarassed to talk about our values and as a result we tend to accept the criticism of our worst critics." (Cunningham 1984).

In the past, values have not been recognized for their importance in the business world. With the discovery of corporate cultures, however the business world is beginning to realize that the best companies are often companies whose executives pay a lot of attention to corporate values. Ironically, while the business world seems to be discovering the importance of values, we who have a rich tradition of values risk losing ours. If we should surrender the heart and soul of health care, the American public has but one alternative – one our society has been moving away from – that is, to turn to government.

REFERENCES

Connors, Edward J. "Corporate Health Leadership" presented at the 20th Annual National Forum on Hospital and Health Affairs, Duke University, Durham, North Carolina, May 1, 1984.

Cunningham, Robert M. Jr. "Closing the Loop" presented at the 20th Annual National Forum on Hospital and Health Affairs, Duke University, Durham, North Carolina, May 1, 1984.

Ginzberg, Eli. "The Monetarization of Medical Care." *The New England Journal of Medicine*, 310 (18): 1162–1165, May 3, 1984.

Peters, Thomas J. and Waterman, Robert H. *In Search of Excellence.* New York: Warner Brooks Edition, 1984.

Selznick, Philip. *Leadership in Administration.* New York: Harper and Row, 1957.

Sigmond, Robert M. "Social Implications of New Business Strategies for Health Care Corporations" presented at Rush-Presbyterian-St. Lukes Medical Center, Chicago, Illinois, March 1984.

Veatch, Robert M. "Ethical Dilemmas of For Profit Enterprise in Health Care," in *The New Health Care for Profit.* Edited by Bradford H. Gray. Washington, D.C.: National Academy Press, 1983.

Discussion – Access

Dr. Warren Greenberg, *Associate Professor, Department of Health Services Administration, The George Washington University*: Perhaps we should look at the incentives of the nonprofit and for-profit hospitals. I would like to ask a question. We have heard statements today about for-profits having incentives for efficiencies; for not doing procedures when costs exceed benefits; for having sophisticated computer operations; for having quality control. We also hear comments that for-profits have a social commitment, which is somewhat surprising given that I do not see pharmaceutical companies providing free drugs, doctors providing free medical care, construction firms providing free houses, or food companies providing free food.

I would like to ask, then, perhaps Bob or Sam, what are the goals of the for-profit hospital and then, perhaps Phil, as a representative of the nonprofit, or Myles, as a representative of a nonprofit hospital, what are the goals of the nonprofit hospital today?

Dr. Robert Vraciu, *President, Center for Health Studies*: I will speak for HCA. I will not pretend to have discussed such an intimate topic with some of our competitors. If we had to prioritize what it is we are doing, we are in the hospital business which is shifting to being in the health care business, our key objective is basically to do that as well as we can.

We have elected to do it on a taxable basis with investor owners. That puts certain types of parameters around which we have to do it. If I had to pinpoint the primary thing that we are out to accomplish, it is to provide high quality health care at a reasonable cost.

Mr. Myles Lash, *formerly Executive Director of Hospital Administration, Medical College of Virginia, Richmond, Virginia; currently, National Director of Health Care, Arthur Young and Company*: As an academic health center, our missions are clear. They are to provide support to our teaching and research mission; to attempt to stay on the forefront in the delivery of medical care and the provision of tertiary care; to encourage the advancement of new technology; and for many of us, to attempt to maintain our historical mission in the provision of charity care. I would hasten to add that the ownership issue is only tangentially related to the maintenance of these important missions.

Mr. Philip S. Birnbaum, *Dean for Administrative Affairs, The George Washington University*: I can only echo what Myles said. Teaching hospitals have an odd place inside the University. The University teaches finance and gives degrees but does not own a bank. It does not own a department store, but it gives degrees in marketing. It does not own a court, but it gives degrees in law; and it may not have to *own* a hospital, but it certainly has to have access to a hospital.

Our mission, like Myles', has that academic underpinning, and like Myles, obviously, I do not think the ownership has to be a major segregating factor.

Ms. Ruth Hanft, *Consultant in Health Policy Research, Washington, D.C.*: I do think it makes a difference between these two institutions. MCV is a state university hospital that has a tradition and a mission from the state of caring for the indigent. George Washington University Hospital is a private nonprofit university hospital, and its mission varies slightly, particularly on that latter issue, indigent care.

Mr. Philip Birnbaum: Clearly, that is true.

Ms. Ruth Hanft: This is very clear, and I think that public/private distinction is absolutely essential.

Mr. Myles Lash: I would be concerned about the funding for indigent care as opposed to who owns these institutions.

Ms. Ruth Hanft: Yes, I agree, but I think if you look at his institution and you look at your institution, they do look very different.

Mr. Myles Lash: I certainly agree.

Dr. Bradford Gray, *Senior Professional Associate, Institute of Medicine*: How is indigent care handled in a for-profit chain hospital? I am curious as to what constraints and incentives administrators face. In other words, by what criteria are they evaluated in terms of whether they are going to get a salary increase the next year, whether they are going to get a bonus. Could you talk a little bit about that?

Dr. Robert Vraciu: One, there will be no bonus. We do not have that kind of incentive program. It is a salary increase program. We have a stock option program that is used as compensation based on performance, which really does not end up that way. The decision is left up, in our company, to the administrator. The evaluation of that administrator is going to be based upon an agreement that is reached between he or she and the division vice president that they report to as part of the annual management plan process.

We fully recognize that many of our hospitals are going to lose money. We have hospitals in Tennessee that have a 22 percent bad debt and charity percentage. That is not held against the administrator. The division vice president has the responsibility of knowing enough about the local circumstances, and if that is part of the scenario, then so be it. If that were to jump to 30 percent and the reason was performance, then I suspect you would say the administrator is going to have some difficulties. But it is a case-by-case determination of what will be expected both in a financial and nonfinancial sense.

Mr. Jon Gabel, *Economist, National Center for Health Services Research*: I want to make two methodological comments on the papers. Bob, you statistically controlled for a number of variables, such as number of hospital beds and metropolitan area shared. I think this is one of the problems with our studies about access to care. It assumes that investor-owned system hospitals randomly select where they locate. In fact, there seems to be a clear pattern. Sixty-three percent of the investor-owned hospitals are found in five states: California, Texas, Tennessee, Florida, and Georgia. They tend to locate in suburban areas and in areas where Blue Cross pays on the basis of charges.

There is a reason as to why investor-owned chain hospitals treat so few indigent and Medicaid patients. The chains might treat similar numbers of these patients as do other area hospitals, but they seek out growing middle class areas. There are lots of financially troubled hospitals in Brownsville or South Bronx or Harlem, but those are not the kind of hospitals you wish to acquire.

Dr. Robert Vraciu: It would be illegal. The State of New York does not permit corporate ownership of hospitals in New York.

Mr. Jon Gabel: In response to the questions on access, Steve, a fundamental problem in measurement is that we can count who gets into the hospital, but we have a difficult time counting who is turned away or who is deterred from entering the hospital. In your survey, should you focus on this issue?

Dr. Stephen Shortell, *A. C. Buehler Distinguished Professor of Hospital and Health Services Management, Northwestern University*: The only comment I would make about that is, in order to get a handle on it, you need to go to a community-based approach to find out who is going where and who is not getting access when they need it. One needs to take a comprehensive look at access and not just in terms of hospital admissions. It is very difficult to do this kind of research.

Dr. James LoGerfo, *Professor of Medicine and Health Services, University of Washington*: I have two comments. One is a residual issue from this morning on the teaching question. Dick Egdahl commented that perhaps we should give house staff more time in different settings, such as outpatient clinics or community hospitals. I think our ability to do that has changed drastically in the last few years. We occasionally get offers by hospitals in our area to expand our residency program. We used to be able to say that if we assign a resident to cover an intensive care unit, we expect some extra support so that we can provide a balanced program for that resident in other settings. We do not get those kinds of balanced requests anymore. Rather, we get requests for the intensive care unit coverage, but not for ambulatory services. I do think our voluntary hospitals are willing to give us residency stipends to subsidize training in ambulatory care. I think that the ability to do that on the part of academic hospitals has changed drastically in the last five years.

Secondly, it is interesting to me in the experience, in terms of funding of the indigent care in Louisville, that they probably struck a deal that any of us who are in the business of providing indigent care would have loved to have but could not. Specifically they said let's start at current base and then just inflate it. The reality has been in most places that dollars for that kind of indigent care did not increase with inflation.

Ms. Judy Miller-Jones, *Director, National Health Policy Forum:* I do not believe it is simply a question of for-profit/nonprofit, but rather a question of indigent care and how various players interpret or follow the rules of the game. We seem to be blaming certain people for playing by the rules and winning at them better than others. But perhaps we should look at the rules of the game that make certain kinds of institutions immediate winners and therefore much more attractive as businesses than others.

I think that the chart you put up showing people's willingness to say that health care is a right is at the crux of this debate. I would like to note a political reality here, for I am not sure that if you asked the question a different way that you would get the same answer. Asking that question the way you phrased it–"Do you believe that the same level of health care should be provided to all people?"–drew a positive reponse of 84 percent. If you ask the same people the question, "would you be willing to have your taxes increased to make sure that the same level of care is provided to all?" Most people would probably lie a bit and say yes. But you have to watch and see if they would be willing to vote for the person who said he was going to raise their taxes to do that. Such a candidate does not usually get elected today, whether at a federal level, a state level, or at a county level.

When we actually look at how people are voting with their feet, I am not sure we can say that people are willing to vote for equal care for all. In fact, when we look across the states, we see it is a rare state that has tried to increase benefits, at least until it has made a great deal of cost savings.

What most of us seem to want to do first is figure out how to take the same level of dollars and spread them farther. States are getting quite imaginative about this, but there is still a feeling that we need to get the fat out of the system and maybe even figure out cheaper ways of providing care.

Ultimately, the question is whether the public will be willing to pay for Barney Clark type of care for indigents. I do not think so. If someone wants to pay for it on their own, that would be okay. But I think we have to force those issues into the public domain. That is what this conference is all about.

We have not yet seen, too many politicians who are willing to say these things publicly. Some policy people and some academics are saying them, and that is all to the good. But you do not see too many politicians who are willing to say ask the public what level of care they are willing to vote for and pay for.

Dr. Gary Filerman, *President, AUPHA*: Steve, I am a little concerned about your initial profile of, or statement of, the problem of access. It seems to me that The Robert Wood Johnson Foundation Reports have been giving a different answer to that question. Or is it the plateauing point that you are making primarily, as opposed to them talking about the trend in the reduction of the problem of access? If I understand them correctly, they are saying that there have been, subgroup by subgroup, substantial improvements.

Dr. Stephen Shortell: If you look at the more recent data, essentially not only has there been a plateauing relative to other groups, depending on the indicators you want to choose, they are no better off than 10–15 years ago. Some of the data that Blendon and Rogers have used comes from the same studies that I am referring to. I am not denying that there has been some improvement on some indicators. But when one adjusts even crudely for the differences in health status, differences remain between the poor and other groups.

Ms. Helen Darling, *Director, Human Resources Studies, Government Research Corporation*: I wish to make two comments. First of all, I agree with everything that Judy said. I do not know if it is because we sit in the same sorts of places, but I certainly agree with her. The second is I think we are going to have, sooner than some of us appreciate, more information about differences, and we may not be able to interpret it any better. As we moved to a national pricing system, it is not going to be all gloom and doom; a lot of hospitals in this country will be doing better under the new system than they have ever done. Unless Congress decides to take back, which it probably will try, what it is supposed to give them, those hospitals will have an opportunity to either expand services and community philanthropy. Also, I think businesses do a lot of philanthrophy; people give away a lot of money, and even food stores give away food. They do it after they have made their profits, but nonetheless they do do it.

I think we will begin to see, for example, if a Bartlesville, Oklahoma, nonprofit hospital does something different with this money than the HCA or the AMI hospital down the street. We are going to begin to see those sorts of things, so we will have some very interesting research.

Dr. Stephen Shortell: I would like to make a brief comment. I think for the first time we are going to find out who the good clinicians really are in this country and who the good hospital managers really are, because under this kind of environment, we no longer have the luxury of ordering every test in the book. Up to now, the environment has been relatively benign. We are now going to find out what excellence in management and excellence in being a good clinician is all about.

Ms. Ruth Hanft: I think we have a problem with certain high cost tertiary services being underpriced and certain simpler services being overpriced in the DRG.

Dr. Stephen Shortell: I agree with that.

Ms. Ruth Hanft: So, I am not sure. It may turn out that your academic health centers, even the best and most efficient, such as the University of Pennsylvania, look terrible.

Dr. Stephen Shortell: I would agree with that. I am saying, even among the academic health science centers, you are going to find some that really are going to rise to the forefront and some are not.

Dr. Steve Eastaugh, *Associate Professor, Department of Health Services Administration, the George Washington University*: I want to address this question to Steve Shortell. I think Helen is definitely right with the letters PPS; prospective payment system can either stand for potential poverty system or potential profit system, depending on how you operate. One area of research that I think would be particularly fruitful for an organizational theorist is that the chains seem to not be in any sense homogeneous. There is a lot of heterogeneity between them. In other words, there are some firms that have a higher payout ratio, above 15 percent, to their stockholders. To give one other example, I want to go beyond how chains treat their shareholders and consider such things as the widely varied incentive compensation systems they set up with their managers. That tells you a little bit about their spirit and their values, if you will. In other words, some incentives have to be abandoned when the managers tend to be more interested in short-term incentive pay and less interested in long-run productivity. What do you think about the heterogeneity among the investor-owneds?

We have talked all day as if there is this one thing called the investor-owneds and that they all behave the same.

Dr. Stephen Shortell: I think there is no question about it. As I suggested earlier, there will probably be much greater within-group variation than between-group variations. The systems have different founding roots, different points on the learning curve in regard to their experience, and so forth. They have somewhat different philosophies and cultures. It is also true on the not-for-profit side.

I think you are absolutely right, and all I am saying is we do not know very much about that yet. We have one study now, at Northwestern, which is funded by the National Center for Health Services Research and the Robert Wood Johnson Foundation. In that study we are trying to examine the issue in a way that will be useful to the industry at large. Ownership alone is a poor proxy measure for how the organization will behave. We are studying the underlying strategies of the systems regarding diversification, new product development, marketing, and selected factors. We will be examining how these are associated with differences in performance in regard to cost, profitability, access, and quality. Two years from now we hope to have some answers or at least insights into many of the questions being raised today.

Index

A

Ablow, K., 30
Abrams, Herbert, 80, 83
academic medical center, viii, 20, 21, 22, 24, 25, 28, 29, 30, 47, 52, 53
access, x, 11, 12, 13, 17, 21, 24, 26, 27, 35, 40, 42, 49, 51, 53, 66, 73, 87, 94, 95, 101, 102, 103, 106, 108, 109, 110, 116, 118, 120, 122, 123, 124, 129, 130, 131, 132, 133, 134, 135, 136, 139, 148, 152, 154, 156, 158
access to care, x, xi, 40, 64, 73, 129, 130, 132, 133, 134, 136, 139, 148, 153
access to health care, x, 102, 106, 123, 124, 128
Aday, L.A., 129, 130, 139
adjusted rate, 69
Alexander, Jeffrey, 77, 78, 83, 84
American Hospital Association (AHA), 61, 77, 110
American Medical Association (AMA), 4, 6, 35, 43, 61, 74, 78
American Medical International (AMI), viii, ix, 6, 8, 23, 49, 76, 81, 85
Andersen, R., 129, 130, 139
Association of Academic Health Centers, 33, 34, 37, 42, 43
Association of American Medical Colleges, 5, 6, 36, 42, 43
availability (of supply of health resources and services), 106, 107, 110, 123, 130

B

Basic services, 110, 111
benefit-cost, 101
Bergen, Stanley, 35, 38, 42
Berry, Ralph E., 110, 111
Birnbaum, P.S., viii, 7, 47, 51, 54, 151, 152
Blue Cross, x, 101, 102, 103, 154, 162
Blue Sheet, 5
The Boston Globe, 31
Bowles, L.T., 9, 11, 29, 30
Bradham, D.D., 134, 139
Bromberg, Michael, 42
Brook, Robert, 66, 74, 81, 83
Brown, B.W., 64, 74
Brown, David, 81, 83
Brown, K.J., 135
Brown, Sarah S., 43

Bryant, Rodney, 116, 126
Bunker, J.P., 66, 74, 136, 140
Burnham, John, 82, 83
Burr, Francis H., 7, 18, 30

C

Caper, Philip, 82, 83
case management, 79
case mix, 34, 35, 36, 38, 42, 69, 80
case-mix severity, 69
Centers of Excellence, 22, 29, 35
chain hospitals, 110, 111, 154
Chen, P.M., 69, 75
Clark, M., 22, 30
Codman, E.A., 76, 77, 83
community-wide access, 123
Connors, Edward, 149, 150
cost-based reimbursement, 4, 78, 101
cost-containment, 133, 138
cost-effectiveness, 32, 79
cost-reduction strategies, 66
Council of Teaching Hospitals, 5, 18, 31, 35, 36, 42, 118
county hospitals, 110, 134
Creighton University, 8, 23, 24, 39
Cummins, R.O., 74
Cunningham, Robert, 30, 32, 43, 149, 150

D

Dallek, G., 134, 139
Darr, K., ix, 57
Davis, K., 129, 139
Derzon, Robert A., 65, 69, 71, 74, 117, 126
DeVries, William, 5, 22, 23, 29
diagnosis-related groups (DRG), 5, 38, 78, 79, 81, 102, 103
Diener, Royce, 6
Directory of Accredited Residency Programs, 5
Donabedian, Avedis, 58, 59, 62, 66, 74
Dorwart, R., 142
Doubilet, Peter, 80, 83
DRG (diagnosis-related groups), 5, 38, 78, 79, 81, 102, 103

E

East Tennessee Medical School, 37
Ebert, Robert, 38, 43
economic market incentives, 78, 79
Egdahl, R.H., viii, 19, 45, 51, 52, 87, 97, 156
Emory University, 36
Enthoven, A.C., 66, 74, 136, 140
Ermann, Dan, 4, 6, 132, 134, 139
Ewy, W., 74
expanded revenue base, 24

F

FAH Review, 23, 30, 126
Fanara, Philip, 102, 104
Feder, Jith, 34, 43
Fishman, Linda E., 38, 43
Fitzgerald, John, 122, 123, 126
flagship, 21, 23, 24, 25, 26, 28, 29, 48, 51
Flood, A.B., 69, 74, 87
for-profit chains, viii, 3, 19, 20, 21, 24, 28, 29, 30, 54
for-profit hospitals, vii, viii, ix, x, xi, 3, 5, 7, 33, 35, 58, 65, 68, 69, 70, 71, 77, 90, 92, 101, 102, 103, 151
for-profit medicine, 58
Forrest, W.H., 64, 74
freestanding investor owned chains, 111
Fuchs, Victor R., 80, 83
funding sources, 107

G

Gabel, Jon, 4, 6, 91, 92, 132, 134, 139, 153, 154
Garber, Alan M., 80, 83
George Washington University, vii, viii, ix, x, 3, 7, 8, 11, 46, 47, 52, 59, 95, 101, 151, 152
Gibson, Louis E., 126
Ginzberg, Eli, 30, 31, 33, 43, 78, 83, 146, 150
governance, viii, 9, 12, 14, 17, 18, 38, 39, 77, 148

graduate medical education, viii, 5, 33, 34, 37, 38, 40, 52
Greenberg, W., x, 101, 102, 104, 151

H

Hadley, Jack, 34, 43
Hanft, Ruth, viii, 32, 38, 42, 43, 46, 47, 53, 88, 90, 152, 153, 157
Harvard Medical School, 7, 18, 26, 28, 47, 89
Health Care Financing Review, 116, 126
Health Maintenance Organization, 35, 38, 39, 102
Heyssel, Robert, 33, 43
Hill-Burton hospitals, 109
Hill-Burton requirements, 34
Himmelstein, D.V., 135, 138, 139
Homer, C.G., 134, 139
Horn, Susan D., 38, 43
Hospital Corporation of America (HCA), 7, 26, 28, 29, 31
Humana Corporation, 120
Humana, Inc., 7, 22, 35

I

Iglehart, John, 33, 34, 43
indigent patients, 36, 101, 102, 116, 118, 120, 123, 124
In Search of Excellence, 145, 150
Institutional Differences Study, 64
Institutional Review Board, 23
Inui, T.S., 74
investor-owned, 88, 97, 111, 112
investor-owned chains, 6, 63, 123, 148
investor-owned corporations, 39
investor-owned hospitals, x, 4, 32, 33, 35, 39, 40, 47, 53, 61, 62, 77, 87, 88, 105, 106, 108, 110, 111, 113, 115, 116, 117, 118, 122, 123, 134, 135, 147, 148, 153
investor ownership, 63

J

Joint Commission on Accreditation of Hospitals, 148
joint-ventures, 121
Jones, David, 23

K

Katz, H.M., 69, 74, 134, 140
Kaufman, R.P., vii, 3, 9, 46, 53
Kloss, Linda, 81, 83
Klosterman, R.E., 135, 139
Kmetz, Donald, 7, 18, 25
Knox, Richard, 31, 123, 126

L

Lansing, Allan, 22
leasing, viii, 19, 20, 25, 26, 27, 28
  psychiatric hospital, 26, 27
  university hospital, 23
Lewin, Lawrence S., 65, 69, 71, 74, 117, 126, 134, 139
Light, Donald W., 76, 83
Linzer, Mark, 80, 84
LoGerfo, J.P., ix, 60, 63, 66, 71, 74, 75, 77, 84, 86, 92, 136, 141, 154
Luft, H., 66, 74, 136, 140
Lutheran Hospital and Homes Society, 81, 83

M

Marshall Medical School, 37
Margulies, Rhea, 65, 69, 74, 117, 126
Massachusetts General Hospital, 7, 26, 34
McLean Hospital Corporation, 30
McNaughton, Donald S., 3, 6
McNerney, W.J., 128, 140
Medicaid, 43, 57, 93, 102, 116, 117, 118, 124, 128, 134
medical center, viii, 26, 35, 47
Medical College of Virginia, 36, 93, 152
medical schools, viii, 7, 19, 20, 32, 33, 34, 36, 37, 41, 53
medical staff, ix, x, 4, 13, 60, 61, 62, 71, 72, 77, 78, 115, 116, 145
Medicare, 37, 41, 43, 57, 78, 93, 102, 116, 117, 118, 124, 129, 134
Medicare Advisory Council, 5

Medicare Hospital Trust Fund, 5
monetarization, 78
Moien, M., 60, 62, 74
monitoring systems, 81
Montefiore Hospital, 34
Morrisey, Michael A., 78, 83, 84
Morrison, Rev. Michael, S.J., 24
Mott, Basil, J.F., ix, 88, 90, 91, 93, 95, 143
Moxley, J. H., ix, 9, 11, 12, 49, 60, 61, 76, 85, 86, 87, 88, 89, 90, 91, 93, 94
Mullner, Ross, 118, 120
multi-hospital systems, 4, 60, 117, 118, 144, 148
multi-unit systems, 132, 148
municipal hospitals, 36
Munson, R.C., 38, 43

N

National Conference of State Legislators, 124, 126
national health financing policy issue, 135, 139
National Institutes of Health, 5, 40
The New York Times, 31
non-group individuals, 102
non-profit, 101, 102, 103
non-profit charitable foundation, 29
not-for-profit hospitals, 33, 38, 42, 58, 60, 108, 110, 111, 117, 122

O

obligation contracts, 108
outcome of medical services, 59

P

Palmer, R.H., 64, 74, 77, 84
patient care information, 61, 82
patient mix, 22, 32, 107, 116, 123
Pattison, R.V., 69, 74, 134, 140
Pauly, Mark, 101, 103
peer review, 29, 61, 80
Peters, Thomas, 145, 146, 150
physician presence, 72
physician services, 61, 78, 103, 123
Placek, P.J., 60, 62, 69, 74
Preferred Provider Organization, 38
President's Commission for the Study of Ethical Problems in Biomedical Research, 74
process of medical services, 58, 59
profit-maximizing strategies, 66
profit motive, ix, 57, 76
prospective pricing, 4, 76, 78, 79, 81, 149
prospective reimbursement, 102
public hospitals, 42, 53, 69, 78, 88, 90, 96, 97, 102, 110, 117, 118, 129, 134, 136, 138

Q

quality care, 57, 59, 76, 77, 80, 82, 83

R

Raine, G., 30
rationing, 72, 129, 130, 131, 132
Redisch, Michael, 101, 103
Rehm, S.M., 75
Reilly, C., 74, 77, 84
Reilly, M., 74, 77, 84
Relman, Arnold S., 7, 18, 30, 31, 32, 43, 101, 103, 104, 105, 126
research, vii, ix, xi, 3, 4, 5, 6, 8, 11, 12, 17, 18, 19, 20, 21, 22, 23, 25, 26, 27, 28, 29, 30, 32, 33, 35, 37, 38, 40, 41, 48, 50, 60, 61, 77, 78, 79, 81, 82, 85, 91, 94, 95, 132, 134, 136, 151, 154, 157
Roeder, P.C., ix, 60, 61, 76
Roth, Amy, 35, 38, 42
Rushefsky, M., 134, 139

S

St. Joseph's Hospital, 8, 23
St. Vincent's Hospital, 81
Schlesinger, M., 134, 140
Schott, W. R., 74
scope of services, 110, 113, 130, 134
Selznick, Philip, 146, 150
service mix, 108, 110, 115, 123, 138

severity group, 81
Shaw, Selm H., 109, 126
Shortell, Stephen, x, 71, 75, 77, 78, 83, 84, 102, 103, 128, 132, 136, 140, 141, 154, 156, 157, 158
Sigmond, Robert, 145, 149, 150
Silverman, James F., 83
Sloan, Frank, 32, 43, 113, 117, 118, 120, 127, 134, 141
Smith, Thomas C., 34, 35, 44, 105
Stanford University Medical Center, 80
structure of medical services, 58
Subcommittee on Health and the Environment, 126
Symbion, 23, 29

T

Taffel, S., 60, 62, 74
teaching hospitals, 19, 20, 32, 33, 34, 35, 36, 37, 38, 39, 40, 41, 42, 47, 48, 53, 54
Tax Equity Fiscal Responsibility Act (TEFRA), 149
Tosteson, D.C., 7, 18
Townsend, J., 135, 141
Tulane University, 36
two-tier system of care, 130

U

uncompensated care, 34, 36, 37, 42, 48, 53, 96, 97, 117, 118, 120, 122, 123, 124, 134, 135
undergraduate clinical education, 37
(unfunded) clinical research, 35
unprofitable customers, 149
University of Louisville, 7, 8, 22, 25, 29, 39, 120
University of Southern Florida, 27
University of Utah, 5, 22, 23
University Psychiatric Center, Inc., 27, 31
utilization review, 102

V

Valvona, Joseph, 118, 121, 127
Veatch, Robert, 147, 150
vertical systems, 73
Veteran's Administration, 36
voluntary, 12, 57, 69, 73, 88, 90, 97, 134, 138, 148
voluntary hospitals, 42, 69, 88, 90, 95, 110, 111, 113, 118, 134, 148, 154
voluntary system hospital, 132, 134, 135, 136, 138, 139, 148
Vraciu, Robert, x, 32, 43, 102, 103, 108, 117, 118, 127, 134, 141, 151, 153, 154

W

The Wall Street Journal, 31
Waterman, Robert, 145, 146, 150
Watt, J.M., 71, 74
Weick, Karl, 145
Wheeler, J.R. C., 74
Williams, R.L., 65, 69, 71, 75, 140
Wright State Medical School, 37
Wyszewianski, L., 74

Z

Zubcoff, Michael, 82, 83